D0968216

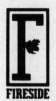

FIRESIDE

Joel R. Saper, M.D., and
Kenneth R. Magee, M.D.

FREEDOM FROM HEADACHES

A Personal Guide for
Understanding and Treating
Headache, Face, and Neck Pain

REVISED and UPDATED

A FIRESIDE BOOK
Published by Simon & Schuster
New York London Toronto Sydney Tokyo Singapore

First Fireside Edition, 1981
Published by Simon & Schuster, Inc.
Simon & Schuster Building
Rockefeller Center
1230 Avenue of the Americas
New York, New York 10020

FIRESIDE and colophon are trademarks of Simon & Schuster, Inc.
Designed by Irving Perkins

Manufactured in the United States of America

15   16   17   18   19   20

Library of Congress Cataloging in Publication Data

Saper, Joel R
   Freedom from headaches.

   (A Fireside book)
   Includes index.
   1. Headache–Prevention.   2. Pain–Prevention.
I. Magee, Kenneth R., joint author.   II. Title.
RC392.S36   1980   616'.047   79-26364

ISBN 0-671-25404-9

ACKNOWLEDGMENTS

To our secretary and typist, Ms. Diana Berry, for her immense patience, skill, and devoted effort to this book. If she has not, by now, developed headaches from the many retypings of this manuscript, she never will.

To Mr. William Sauber of Midland, Michigan, an author and monosodium glutamate-sensitive headache sufferer, for his interest in our work and for his generous sharing of his experiences and scientific references.

To Drs. Arnold Friedman, John R. Graham, Seymour Diamond, Donald J. Dalessio, Leonard L. Loveshin, Robert Kunkel, Lee Kudrow, John Edmeads, James Dexter, Otto Appenzeller, Ninan Mathew, William Speed, Russell Packard, Neil Raskin, and Robert E. Ryan, Sr., and the many other internationally known clinicians, researchers, and headache authorities whose scientific studies and observations have made writing this book possible.

*To the thousands of headache sufferers
who have come to us in pain—
for all that they have taught us about headaches,
human nature, and compassion.*

A PERSONAL NOTE

During the final days of this manuscript's completion, my father, Leonard Saper, died unexpectedly at the age of fifty-seven. His ever-present encouragement and support will always be remembered. My contribution to this book, which he so proudly and eagerly awaited, reflects his influence.

JOEL R. SAPER, M.D.

Contents

11

The Headache Ordeal: An Introduction and History

"I feel as though a vise were squeezing my brain out."
"My head is splitting open."
"It feels as though a machine were grinding my head to pieces."
"It feels as though a hot iron were pressed to my temples."
"My head hurts so much I know I must have a brain tumor."
"A spike is being driven through my head."
"It's as though I were wearing a hat five sizes too small."
"If you can't stop these headaches, I'm going to commit suicide."

More than thirty million people in the United States suffer the incapacitating agony of recurring head pain. Although nearly everyone has experienced a headache at some time, and despite centuries of medicine's recording of the details of this condition, the mysteries of the headache problem continue to defy a complete understanding. Neither the exact cause nor any consistently reliable treatment is currently within the immediate grasp of scientific knowledge. It is curious indeed that a medical condition of such magnitude, disabling influence, and long history should remain so shrouded in myth, misinformation, and mystery.

The impact of frequent and severe headaches is as extraordinary as it is underestimated. Many headache victims suffer not only discomfort but also the frustrations and isolation that accompany recurring and incapacitating pain.

Lewis Carroll, author of *Alice's Adventures in Wonderland* and *Through the Looking-Glass*, suffered from headaches. Through the character of Tweedledum, Lewis Carroll states, " 'I'm very brave, generally, only today I happen to have a headache.' " As suggested by the loss of Tweedledum's courage, recurring headaches can have a devastating impact on the lives of those who suffer from frequent head pain. Marital discord, depression, fear, isolation, drug abuse, a feeling of helplessness, and even suicide are only a few of the consequences characterizing a headache-possessed existence.

Head pain is not like other pain. A headache occurs at the center of the mind; it affects the captain of the ship and disrupts the control center of the body. Headaches do not simply strike at your muscles or organs; they attack the very essence of you. Those of you who have experienced a truly severe headache know that when the head aches, the entire body suffers. Fear that head pain stems from a serious or life-threatening condition adds to the anxieties and frustrations that plague the victim.

A bad headache is not demonstrable like a cast on a broken wrist or stitches zippering up a recent surgical incision, and many doubting and skeptical persons question the integrity of anyone complaining of frequent pain, particularly when no visible proof of injury is present. The tolerance commanded by less disabling symptoms, like a sore throat or a stomach ache, is typically lacking if you miss work and use a headache as the excuse. For the victim with recurring nighttime headaches, the statement "Not tonight, darling, I've got a splitting headache" is most often not simply the ballad of an unwilling partner, but the pleading of a truly disabled participant who is deprived of much more in life than enjoyable lovemaking.

Perhaps no other condition affecting so many people so disrupts the lives of its victims and yet evokes so little sympathy and compassion for the afflicted. Few other victims of legitimate disease are subjected to as much skepticism regarding their symptoms.

As the headache patient suffers frustration and pain, there comes an irresistible temptation to resort to tantalizing offerings of help from unscientific and medically illegitimate sources. Perhaps more than any other patient, the headache victim is prey both to advertisements claiming relief of pain and to modern-day medical charlatans selling their "miracle headache cures." But, alas, after visiting countless physicians, taking enormous quantities of pills, and even trying unconventional means of finding pain relief, the victim still endures recurring head pain.

Those of you who have lived many years suffering from headaches should take some comfort in knowing that you are among an exclusive group of fellow headache sufferers. The list of famous headache sufferers is quite impressive and includes such notable individuals as Cervantes, Thomas Jefferson, Sigmund Freud, Ulysses S. Grant, Karl Marx, Julius Caesar, Leo Tolstoy, Virginia Woolf, Edgar Allan Poe, Lewis Carroll, Tchaikovsky, Chopin, Charles Darwin, and George Bernard Shaw. These notables, like you, experienced the agony and limitations imposed by this disabling affliction. And, like many of you, they persevered day by day to overcome the disability.

The history of headache predates recorded time. Small holes found drilled in the skulls of prehistoric human remains may well have represented attempts at relieving pain and suggest the possibility that headaches plagued our earliest ancestors. Trephining the skull, drilling small holes through the bones, remains today as a neurosurgical technique for diagnosing and treating certain conditions and for relieving abnormally high pressure inside the skull. Our understanding and treatment of headaches have progressed considerably from that time, although no one would dispute that we still have a long way to go.

Dr. Arnold Friedman, formerly of New York City and now of Arizona, is a world-famous headache authority who has devoted a major portion of his life to furthering our understanding of headache and its treatment. In addition to his world-renowned scientific contributions to the field, Dr. Friedman has researched the history of headache and the wide-ranging therapies imposed on headache sufferers. His writings provide many references to these early treatments, some of which still remain in the folklore and wives' tales that surround the subject of headache.

While in some respects our present approach to headaches remains somewhat primitive, if you have suffered uncomfortable adverse side effects from "modern" treatments you might find it soothing to learn how our ancestors were treated for their headaches.

Early therapy often reflected strong religious influences and included long pilgrimages to famous shrines. One rather popular cure, described in an Irish manuscript, instructed the headache sufferer to pray to the eye of Isaiah, tongue of Solomon, mind of Benjamin, heart of St. Paul, and faith of Abraham.

Animals and animal parts were widely employed for headache treatment. One therapy involved placing the skins of reptiles over the face and head. If that did not work, one could attach leeches to the body to induce bleeding and subsequent blister formation on the skin. Another treatment included the use (application or ingestion is not clear) of elder seeds, cow's brain, and goat dung, all dissolved in vinegar. Still another attempted to soothe the aching head with beaver testes bottled in spirits. Interestingly, it has been shown subsequently that parts of the beaver's genitalia contain salicylate (aspirin).

An English technique for relieving headache consisted of applying dried and powdered flies in a mixture of vinegar to the affected area until blisters developed. The blisters were then punctured in order to allow the "evil humours" to escape. A Mexican therapy consisted of stroking the forehead with a live toad. One therapy included hanging the head of a dead buzzard from the neck of the headache sufferer.

Those compassionate souls who wished to spare animals from the treatment program could apply a metallic object to the painful area and stand for long periods with a noose around their neck. If this failed, one could wrap around the neck a paper soaked in vinegar.

A rather innovative technique was to scrape algae or moss from a statue and hang it from the headache sufferer's neck by a red string. An alternative to this was making an incision in the scalp and applying raw garlic or dill blossoms to the wound. Another variation was to press a hot iron to the head until the original pain lessened.

Though many of these therapies undoubtedly caused more pain than did the headache that they were designed to treat, it should be recognized that many of these were intended to scare the "evil spirits" from the head. Early theories of illness were often based on the belief that it was the body's inhabitation by demons and malevolent forces that accounted for human disease.

We must not regard our ancestors too harshly for their methods of treating headaches. Perhaps someday we too will be judged for our methods of diagnosing and treating disease. It will take considerable charity by future generations to look kindly on some of our "modern" treatment programs. After all, swallowing pills, cutting open skulls and abdomens, and inserting plastic tubes into every conceivable body opening seem frightfully primitive, even by our own present standards and perspectives.

It is from a sensitivity to the headache dilemma that we have written this book. Our aim is to teach you about your disorder, help you to understand the medical approach to pain, make you an informed and discriminating medical consumer, and assist you in helping yourself obtain the safest and most effective means of alleviating your discomfort.

We caution you in the strongest terms not to use the information in this book to indulge in self-diagnosing your own headache problem. Even the most qualified physician is incapable of satisfactorily evaluating or treating his or her own illness, particularly a condition as complex and poorly understood as headaches. NOTHING can substitute for objective and experienced medical care.

This book is, for the most part, neither theory nor speculation. The information it contains is accepted and scientifically founded medical information, supplemented and highlighted with examples and case histories from our own professional experience. We trust that you will use this book wisely to assist you in finding a competent physician, monitor the care you receive, and enable you to reject the unfounded, deceptive, and often dangerous practices to which you are exposed.

Before entering into a discussion of the complex subject of headache pain, we would like to introduce you to the specialty of neurology, since you may be uncertain about this specialty's role in headache care. Neurology is the field of medicine concerned with the functions and disorders of the brain, spinal cord, and the related nerves. Diseases of muscle have also traditionally come under the domain of the neurologist.

Among the more common or well-known neurological disorders are strokes, Parkinson's disease, epilepsy, multiple sclerosis, and muscular dystrophy. Because of the neurologist's interest in disorders of brain function, a neurologist also evaluates impairment of thinking, memory, learning, and verbal expression, as well as those conditions causing coma and pain. It is this broad involvement with diseases of the brain, as well as the origin and treatment of painful conditions, that explains the neurologist's interest in the subject of headache.

Some people use the term "nerves" when referring to symptoms of anxiety and tension. Because a neurologist is involved with the other kind of nerves—strands of tissue that carry messages between the brain and other parts of the body—some of our would-be patients have found themselves at the wrong specialist's door. One prospective patient seeking help for anxiety asked one of us, after he was referred to a psychiatrist, "If I've got a problem with my nerves and you're a nerve doctor, why do I need a psychiatrist?"

A psychiatrist's primary role concerns disturbances of behavior that are not associated with observable physical changes in the brain. A neurologist may be involved with persons having abnormal behavior if physical changes in the brain are possibly responsible for the behavioral abnormalities. Understandably, the two specialties overlap considerably. This is reflected by certification standards that require both psychiatrists and neurologists to demonstrate competence in the alternative specialty.

The term "neuropsychiatrist" was once used to describe a physician who practiced both neurology and psychiatry. However, with a greater understanding of the brain, the mind, and behavior and with the proliferation of enormous amounts of new information about the way the brain functions, it became necessary for those physicians practicing neuropsychiatry to "specialize" in one field or another. Ironically, with even better understanding of the brain and its functions, we are now learning that chemical and physical abnormalities may indeed explain some "psychiatric" disorders. It is quite possible that in the future the differences that now separate the two specialties will again become less distinct.

JOEL R. SAPER, M.D.
KENNETH R. MAGEE, M.D.

Chapter 1 Pain and Its Treatment

Aristotle called pain the passion of the soul, and those of you who have suffered from intense and recurring pain know very well how deeply it erodes the framework of your existence, touching every part of your life. Headache, unlike most other afflictions, has the devilish capacity to begin in childhood and become a lifelong companion. Having headaches can become part of your personality, a characteristic of your very being and identity. Because of this and because the pain and its causes remain a mystery, it is understandable that treating long-standing and recurring pain is neither simple nor straightforward. Chronic headaches are often difficult to treat.

Before entering into a discussion of the various types of headaches and the many important issues concerning headache pain and its treatment, it is appropriate to introduce you to the complex subject of pain itself, along with the many ways that it can be treated.

Psychological elements contribute significantly to pain and its treatment. Although it is not clearly understood just how, the mind exerts an extraordinary influence on the recognition and meaning attached to painful sensations. For example, it may not be until the end of the day that an injury you incurred during an earlier enjoyable activity is felt as pain. But the pain caused by banging a shin on a coffee table while racing to answer a relentlessly ringing telephone hurts immediately and exquisitely.

Other features related to pain also remain obscure. How much do social, emotional, and cultural influences affect your ability to cope with and display your painful experiences? Some families, and even entire cultures, place a very high premium on a stoic toleration of pain and seek to minimize the expression of discomfort. Other cultures encourage the demonstration of suffering, and patterns for the display of pain become part of that culture's personality.

These psychological and cultural factors, together with important biological considerations, ultimately affect how you feel pain by influencing your *pain threshold.* The pain threshold can be described in simple terms as a biological thermostat. When the thermostat is set high, a strong, unpleasant stimulus is required for you to feel pain. When the thermostat is lowered, a mildly unpleasant sensation will be experienced as pain.

The pain threshold varies from person to person and can even change within the same person, depending upon emotional and biological factors. Depression, anxiety, and frustration seem to lower the pain threshold, while happiness, contentment, and enjoyable moments raise it.

Before going further, consider the following questions, which are designed to prime your awareness of a few features of your own personality. Keep the responses to these questions in mind as you read through the book. Understanding yourself is very important when attempting to come to grips with the problem of pain.

Are you a happy person?
Are you irritable without reasonable cause?
Do you like yourself?
Is your life reasonably settled and organized?
Does your life have a goal?
Do you have a bad temper?
Are you an angry person or do you carry a "chip on your shoulder"?

Are you kind and forgiving?
Do you carry grudges?
Are you bored and restless?
Would you like yourself if you saw yourself as others do?
Are you depressed or blue much of the time?
Must you prove your virility or femininity?
Are you dependable?
Do you abuse yourself?
Are you selfish to others?
Do you know how to relax and enjoy life?
Do you try to see the best in every circumstance or prefer to pick out the worst?
Do you tend to blame others for your plight?
Do you feel victimized by life?

Related to the psychological and emotional factors involved in treatment of pain is yet another very important and intriguing phenomenon called the *placebo response.* The word "placebo" translated from Latin means "I will please." A placebo therapy has no established scientific rationale for any benefit it may evoke. The placebo response is the real benefit that comes from such a tablet or capsule. More than 40 percent of people with headaches may have a beneficial response to a placebo treatment. This means that in a group of one hundred patents given a placebo—usually a pill or other treatment with no active therapeutic ingredient—approximately forty will experience at least a temporary improvement.

It is not known with certainty how a "sugar pill" or other therapy that has no currently known scientific basis for effectiveness is able to help some patients feel better. The placebo response may be related to the desire to improve and to the suggestion by a physician or therapist that a particular treatment is of value. Later in this chapter, you will read about substances called *endorphins.* Endorphins are made in the brain and have a remarkable similarity to morphine, a narcotic analgesic. One recent report has suggested that the level of these naturally occurring "pain killers," the endorphins, may rise in the brain of some patients experiencing benefit from a placebo treatment.

An article from the Mayo Clinic entitled "Who Responds to Sugar Pills"* offered an explanation for the placebo response. The report suggested that it is a form of "self-hypnosis" that is particularly effective in certain individuals. Those most likely to have a beneficial placebo response were people who welcomed important responsibilities and liked to act independently. By contrast, the test group of people with the least number of responsibilities, and who had the greatest dependence upon others, was less benefited by a placebo. This study, published prior to the recent work with endorphins, raises the possibility that people of an independent and strong-willed nature may actually have a greater power to control their own physiology than those who do not respond to placebos.

The placebo response is only one of the factors that must be considered in any research study whose goal is to establish the effectiveness of a particular medication. To ensure that the conclusions of any drug study are scientifically valid, the research project must take into account emotional considerations and biases that can affect either the patient or the investigator. These factors must be prevented from influencing the research study. If they are not, the conclusions of the study cannot be considered reliable.

To ensure scientific objectivity, specially designed research techniques are used. One method uses randomly chosen volunteer patients who have similar symptoms. These patients are divided into two groups; one of the groups is given the medication that is to be evaluated and the other group receives a placebo. The patients are not told to which group they belong, and all tablets or capsules are identical in appearance.

A further requirement is that the investigator evaluating the patients' response to the pills does not know to which group the patients belong. This insures against the influence of the investigator's own biases, which are usually unintentional and unknown but can affect the interpretation of the test results. This research technique is referred to as a "double blind" study because neither the patients nor the interpreting investigator knows which patients are receiving which therapy.

* C. G. Moertel, W. F. Taylor, A. Roth, and F. A. J. Tyce, "Who Responds to Sugar Pills," in *Mayo Clinic Proceedings* (February 1976), p. 96.

By studying a treatment in this way, a reasonably objective evaluation can be achieved. If the data obtained from the study suggest a significant difference in effectiveness between the real medication and the placebo, the drug under study is considered more effective than a placebo. This is important because all medications, even ineffective ones, must be considered at least potentially harmful, and a physician must decide which medications possess sufficient potential benefit for their potential risks. Many nonprescription medications, as well as many medicines that require a prescription, do not demonstrate a therapeutic benefit greater than can be achieved with a placebo.

Government agencies have not consistently or effectively acted in the public's interest, so the consumer must sometimes take the time to think about and challenge the deceptive inferences of advertisers selling potentially hazardous and expensive medications, often no more effective than the inexpensive aspirin they contain. The consumer must take the same wary attitude toward the peddlers of unscientific, untested, and sometimes dangerous therapies. Because many headaches and many other painful disorders will eventually subside without any treatment, it is apparent that almost any therapy can initially appear beneficial, irrespective of its actual value or potential adverse effects.

We have started this chapter on the treatment of headaches with this commentary to help you develop a discriminating attitude regarding unscientifically tested and deceptively advertised medicines. You should be equally suspicious of miracle cures or other unusual treatments. Qualified physicians will consider the risks of any therapy, the transiency of many symptoms, and the important emotional contributions that play a role in the patient's response to various therapies before prescribing any medication. You, the consumer, must understand these issues too.

MEDICATION FOR TREATING HEADACHE

There are many different drugs that can be used to treat a headache, and most of these can be placed in one of three categories:

Analgesics,
Mood-altering drugs, and
Specialized drugs that act against the actual cause of the head-
ache.

A physician must decide whether to approach your discomfort by
the abortive, "symptomatic," method (trying to stop a headache
once the symptoms have already begun) or by the preventive
method (trying to prevent the onset of the headache by treating
you daily, similar to the principle concerning the use of birth
control pills).

The abortive, or symptomatic, approach treats the headache
once it has begun. An example would be taking two aspirin when
you feel a headache beginning. While often successful, and relatively simple to use, a major disadvantage of the abortive approach
is that it usually requires the use of drugs that should not be taken
too often. If your head pain occurs more than three or four times
per week, the abortive approach may be medically inappropriate,
since very strong medications are often required for relief with this
method. Another disadvantage of the abortive approach is that
once a bad headache has already begun, even the most potent
medications may not relieve the pain.

The preventive approach is based on the presumption that patients with recurring pain have a certain biological or emotional
predisposition that leads to the development of the discomfort. The
preventive method of treatment is aimed at altering those factors
before the pain develops.

The preventive approach is most often used when the headaches
are frequent and occur with regularity. The medicines used in
the preventive approach are relatively well tolerated when taken
daily. A major disadvantage of the preventive approach is that it
requires the use of medication every day. This is necessary because
there is usually no way to accurately determine on which days the
headache will actually occur. When the headache predictably develops with an event, like a menstrual period or on weekends,
preventive medication can occasionally be used just prior to these
times.

The abortive and preventive approaches can, at times, be used together. For example, if you are placed on a program of preventive therapy but a headache "breaks through," you may be given one of the abortive medications to help relieve that particular headache.

The following are the various categories of medicines used to treat headaches.

Analgesics—Analgesics are medications used to stop pain by raising your pain threshold and in that way reducing the painful experience. Analgesics generally do not affect the cause of the headache but simply lessen the sensation of pain during the period of the medication's effectiveness, usually two to six hours. This type of therapy has the advantage of being simple, but analgesic treatment is not always effective in reducing pain. Most analgesic drugs cannot be taken safely on a daily basis. While mild analgesics, like aspirin, are effective for many headaches, some analgesics—including aspirin—may be capable of injuring organs such as the stomach, liver, and kidneys with prolonged use.

Numerous problems surround the use of analgesics in addition to the above. Some patients experience a "high" feeling from certain analgesics, and this may result in drug abuse and subsequent habituation. Another very real problem created by using analgesics is that they mask pain. Pain is a symptom. It suggests that something is wrong. Covering up the pain before complete evaluation of its cause is determined can be hazardous because the patient and even the physician are deprived of an important reminder that a problem exists and they can be lulled into a false sense of complacency.

Another significant problem regarding the use of analgesics is that daily use may actually intensify your perception of pain after the analgesic is metabolized, about four hours after ingestion. Recent research suggests that this can set up a "rebounding" cycle, requiring continued use of analgesics in order to sustain relief. In other words, while the available data is still sparse, researchers in the field have observed some evidence to suggest that daily use of analgesics may actually enhance, through various chemical reactions, a person's perception of pain. This process may be somewhat similar to the phenomenon observed by many people when an itchy rash is scratched. The itch is a form of pain created by irritation of the nerve endings in the skin. While the nails are scratching the itchy area, the itch is relieved and a pleasurable sensation is experienced. When scratching ceases, the itch may actually become more intense—even painful—than prior to being scratched. It is believed that this phenomenon may represent a "hypersensitization" process, due to irritation of the pain receptors from repeated scratching.

Also related to the regular use of analgesics is the possibility that pain, being a biological reaction, is "trainable," not unlike one's ability to wake up at a customary time each morning. We have all observed that once the body becomes used to a particular function, it will develop a symptom in order to obtain that to which it has become accustomed. For example, if one regularly goes to bed at 11 o'clock each evening, a sense of tiredness will develop around that time. Depending upon the hours that one regularly eats, hunger will intensify as that time approaches. The repetitive use of analgesics may result in a similar relationship. If the body develops a sense of acceptance of daily analgesics and, for one of a variety of poorly understood reasons, begins to depend upon these analgesics, the body will develop a symptom to get that which it seeks—in the case of analgesics, pain.

Analgesics vary in potency, side effects, and cost. They range from simple analgesics, such as aspirin, to narcotic analgesics, like codeine and morphine. A variety of preparations containing one or more analgesics in combination with other drugs, including antihistamines, stimulants, sedatives, nasal decongestants, and antinauseants, are available as prescription and over-the-counter, nonprescription drugs.

Before discussing some specific analgesics, you should know that the dose of one drug is not necessarily equivalent to an equal dose of another drug. For example, 50 milligrams (mg.) of Drug X may be fatal, whereas 500 milligrams (mg.) of Drug Y may be an ideal dose. Also, people differ dramatically in their response to similar doses of the same drug.

Ordinary aspirin is the best and least expensive of the simple analgesics for most painful conditions, including many headaches. In addition to relieving pain, aspirin has these other important properties: the ability to reduce fever, to diminish inflammation, and to lessen blood coagulation. But an overdose of aspirin can be fatal. Adult aspirin tablets contain approximately 325 mg. of acetylsalicylic acid, and the usual adult dose is two tablets taken every four to six hours, as necessary. Aspirin should be avoided or used with caution by patients with certain stomach disorders, like ulcers, or by anyone taking oral antidiabetic preparations or anticoagulants. Anticoagulants are "blood thinners" and thus reduce the ability of the blood to coagulate. Patients with clotting deficiencies must avoid aspirin.

Aspirin, the "ingredient prescribed most by physicians for pain," as many commercial advertisers refer to it, is an excellent drug and is recommended for routine pain relief. We do not believe that the more expensive brands of aspirin, including the buffered aspirin, have substantial advantage over the less expensive "house" brands. Buffering, in simple terms, means counteracting the acidity that may play a role in causing the stomach distress associated with aspirin's use. Sometimes aspirin becomes stale and loses its effectiveness; if your aspirin has a decidedly vinegary taste and smell, it should be discarded for a fresh supply.

An appropriate substitute for aspirin is acetaminophen (Tylenol and Datril). Acetaminophen has analgesic as well as fever-lowering capabilities similar to aspirin. Acetaminophen does not cause some of the side reactions associated with aspirin, but as with other analgesics an abuse can result in liver and kidney abnormalities and even death. An overdose of acetaminophen, particularly in children, may be very serious and more difficult to treat than an overdose of aspirin.

Acetaminophen has the advantage of not irritating the stomach or interfering with anticoagulation therapy, but it lacks aspirin's anti-inflammatory properties, which make aspirin much more effective in the treatment of some of the pain in arthritic conditions. Acetaminophen tablets usually contain approximately 325 mg. of the drug per tablet, and the average dose is the same as the average dose of aspirin, two tablets every four to six hours.

Let's look at a sample of over-the-counter nonprescription "combination of ingredient" preparations. Many of these have gained wide popularity. The medications we shall discuss were chosen simply because they are well known and are probably familiar to most readers. These preparations are more expensive than simple aspirin or acetaminophen, and most of them combine aspirin and/or acetaminophen in various dosages with other less effective analgesics, caffeine, or additional ingredients.

Caffeine is contained in many products used for relief of headache. Caffeine is an extract of plants and seeds from which cola, coffee, cocoa, and tea are derived. Caffeine acts as a mild stimulant and can minimally constrict blood vessels. Caffeine may also assist the absorption of medication from the stomach. These features make caffeine a popular ingredient in headache preparations. But too much caffeine can cause jitteriness, affect heart rate and blood pressure, and even cause headaches, and we feel its liberal use in these preparations is unwarranted.

Empirin remains a popular headache remedy. Until recently this Burroughs Wellcome product contained aspirin, phenacetin, and caffeine, familiar to many, generically, as APC tablets. Phenacetin has now been removed from the formulation because of reports attributing kidney damage to its use. Caffeine has also been deleted because the reasons for its inclusion in a pain remedy require further scientific validation of efficacy and safety. As currently marketed, Empirin contains only aspirin.

Aspirin or acetaminophen may be compounded with codeine in varying amounts (16 mg., 30 mg., 60 mg.). Such combination analgesics may be purchased as inexpensive generic versions or as brand name products. Thus, Empirin #2 tablets contain 16 mg. of codeine, Empirin #3 contains 30 mg. of codeine, and Empirin #4 contains 60 mg. of codeine. Codeine-containing drugs require a physician's prescription in the United States, but can easily be purchased "over-the-counter" in Canada, a practice that we think is unwise.

Excedrin contains approximately

250 mg. of aspirin,
250 mg. of acetaminophen, and
65 mg. of caffeine.

The amount of acetaminophen contained in each Excedrin tablet (approximately 250 mg.) is about three-quarters the amount in a plain acetaminophen tablet (325 mg.), and the amount of caffeine (64 mg.) is about one-half that of the caffeine in a cup of coffee. The content of aspirin (approximately 250 mg.) is also about three-quarters of that present in one aspirin (325 mg.). So, in all probability, most people can get about the same amount of pain relief from one and a half ordinary low-cost aspirin tablets as from one Excedrin tablet.

Each Vanquish tablet contains approximately

227 mg. of aspirin,
194 mg. of acetaminophen,
33 mg. of caffeine,
dried aluminum hydroxide gel, and
magnesium hydroxide.

(The latter two are "antacids" used for buffering.)

A Vanquish tablet contains less aspirin than a plain aspirin tablet, much less acetaminophen than one acetaminophen tablet, such as Tylenol, and about the amount of caffeine contained in one-third cup of coffee. You could approximate the analgesic effectiveness of one Vanquish tablet by taking one aspirin tablet, one-half an acetaminophen tablet, and drinking one-third cup of coffee along with an antacid.

An Anacin tablet contains

400 mg. of aspirin, and
32 mg. of caffeine.

One Anacin has the analgesic equivalent of about one and one-third ordinary aspirin tablets and a small amount of caffeine. Anacin is advertised as the "medicine with more of the ingredient that doctors recommend most for pain," that ingredient being aspirin. The advertisements and promotions also claim that Anacin contains an "extra ingredient" not found in plain aspirin. This extra ingredient, through the process of elimination, must be caffeine, less than one-third the amount of caffeine contained in a cup of coffee. The recommended dose of Anacin is two tablets every four to six hours. The approximate effectiveness of a single Anacin tab-

Table I Analgesics

Name	Active Ingredients/Tablet (Approximate Contents)	Effect
Aspirin	325 mg. Acetylsalicylic acid	Analgesic Reduces fever Reduces coagulation Reduces inflammation
Tylenol Datril	325 mg. Acetaminophen	{ Analgesic { Reduces fever
Tempra Liquiprin	Liquid form (children)	
Empirin	325 mg. Aspirin	Analgesic*
Excedrin	250 mg. Aspirin 250 mg. Acetaminophen 65 mg. Caffeine	Analgesic Analgesic See text
Vanquish	227 mg. Aspirin 194 mg. Acetaminophen 33 mg. Caffeine Buffers	Analgesic Analgesic See text
Cope	421 mg. Aspirin 32 mg. Caffeine Buffers	Analgesic See text
Anacin	400 mg. Aspirin 32 mg. Caffeine	Analgesic See text
Ascriptin	325 mg. Aspirin Buffers	Analgesic
Bufferin	324 mg. Aspirin Buffers	Analgesic
Percogesic	325 mg. Acetaminophen 30 mg. Phenyltoloxamine	Analgesic Antihistamine (sedative)

* See above for additional effects of aspirin.

Comment	Adult Dose	Effective Practical Alternative (Double for Usual Adult Dose)
Effective for many painful conditions Relatively safe Inexpensive Do not use if have stomach disorder or if using blood thinners or antidiabetic drugs	2 tabs. every 4–6 hours	
Effective for many painful conditions Relatively safe Prolonged use can harm liver	2 tabs. every 4–6 hours See package insert	
Compare cost to plain aspirin or acetamino- phen	2 tabs. every 4–6 hours	1 Aspirin ½ Acetaminophen (Tylenol, Datril) ½ cup brewed coffee
Compare cost to plain aspirin or acetamino- phen	2 tabs. every 4–6 hours	1 Aspirin ½ Acetaminophen ¼ cup brewed coffee Antacid tablet
Compare cost to plain aspirin	2 tabs. every 4–6 hours	
Compare cost to plain aspirin	2 tabs. every 4–6 hours	1½ Aspirin ¼ cup brewed coffee
Compare cost to plain aspirin	2 tabs. every 4–6 hours	1 Aspirin Antacid tablet
Compare cost to plain aspirin	2 tabs. every 4–6 hours	1 Aspirin Antacid tablet
Compare cost to plain aspirin or acetamino- phen	2 tabs. every 4–6 hours	

let can be achieved by taking one and one-half aspirin and drinking one-third cup of strong coffee.

A summary of these and other over-the-counter nonprescription analgesic preparations has been provided for your convenience in comparing the ingredients and action of these drugs. (See Table I, pp. 34–35.) This table also contains a formula for duplicating, less expensively, these drug combinations, using inexpensive aspirin, acetaminophen, and caffeine (caffeine is not essential to the analgesic effectiveness of these agents or alternatives). If you compare prices between the combination drugs and the simple aspirin and acetaminophen that they contain, and add a little extra cost for some caffeine, we think you will be surprised at how disproportionately expensive many of the combination drugs are. An Anacin tablet, for example, which contains only slightly more aspirin than one aspirin plus caffeine, is approximately four times as expensive as a house-brand aspirin tablet.

In Chapter 7 there is a discussion of the treatment of sinus headache. Much of what has been said about the ordinary headache remedies also applies to many of the so-called "sinus headache" tablets. Most of these drugs combine various combinations of analgesics, antihistamines, decongestants, and caffeine.

Antihistamines have a number of medicinal properties. Among these are an "anti-inflammatory" effect, which helps reverse some symptoms of allergic conditions, and a sedative effect. Decongestants are agents that have vasoconstrictive properties and are used in cold and sinus preparations to constrict the blood vessels and membranes of the nose and nasal sinuses.

A Sinarest tablet contains 325 mg. of acetaminophen, 2 mg. of chlorpheniramine maleate (an antihistamine), and 18.75 mg. of phenylpropanolamine (a decongestant). Sine-Off contains 325 mg. of aspirin, 2 mg. of chlorpheniramine maleate (an antihistamine), and 18.75 mg. of phenylpropanolamine (a decongestant). Sine-Aid contains 325 mg. of acetaminophen and 25 mg. of phenylpropanolamine (a decongestant).

Table II contains a list of these and other nonprescription sinus headache remedies along with their ingredients.

We see a number of problems with these actively promoted nonprescription combination sinus headache drugs. Most of them contain an antihistamine. In allergic conditions, antihistamines are useful, but a large percentage of patients with sinus congestion and sinus headaches (see Chapter 5) do not have allergy as a basis for their symptoms, so antihistamines in these instances are of little or no value. The decongestants contained in some of these preparations are poorly absorbed from the stomach when administered in tablet form and are thus relatively ineffective at recommended doses. When taken in excessive amounts, however, these decongestants can raise blood pressure and affect heart rate and circulation to various important organs and, therefore, should not be taken unless absolutely necessary and only after proper medical evaluation.

In general, the nonprescription combination analgesics and sinus headache medications offer a collection of drug ingredients that include aspirin, acetaminophen, and a number of extra ingredients that are of doubtful value for most people who turn to them for relief of their symptoms. Also, when taken in excessive amounts, these ingredients, including caffeine, may have adverse effects upon various body functions.

We doubt that these drugs have any significant benefit other than the effect of the simple aspirin or acetaminophen that they contain. Yet these combination substances are considerably more expensive than an aspirin or an acetaminophen tablet.

We recognize that many people believe that they benefit from these combination drugs, and perhaps some do. But we do not think that the "shotgun" approach to symptoms provided by these combination-of-ingredient drugs is a medically sound way to treat disease. Such an approach forces often misinformed patients to take either unnecessary or potentially hazardous substances for their particular medical condition. (In Chapter 5 we will try to convince you that most people who think they have sinus disease and sinus headaches do not suffer from these problems at all.)

We suspect that many people who believe that they benefit from these drugs are benefiting from the simple analgesics in them and perhaps from some placebo effect as well.

We suggest that patients with pain, particularly head pain, take simple aspirin or acetaminophen in the appropriate dosages with a glass of water and a little light food to help avoid stomach discomfort. If adequate pain relief is not achieved after a reasonable time, medical advice should be sought. Relying on regular or excessive use of these combination tablets exposes you to many potential hazards. Also, as we have already suggested, too much caffeine can actually cause headaches as well as a variety of other symptoms. And keep in mind that the caffeine ingested when you take these medications adds to the caffeine that is in foods and beverages. More about this problem in Chapter 9.

All these warnings about nonprescription combination medications hold true for the prescription combination drugs as well. The mere fact that they require a prescription does not mean that they are effective. A major difference with prescription drugs is that there is a source of accountability and control—your physician. You can ask your doctor about the ingredients in the medication prescribed, the appropriate doses for you, and the potential side effects.

As mentioned earlier in the discussion of the placebo response, recent research suggests that the brain is capable of producing its own "analgesics." These substances have been called endorphins, and they possess a remarkable similarity to morphine, one of the most potent narcotic analgesics. The widespread implications of these findings have not yet been fully appreciated. How the brain relieves its own perception of pain, what mechanisms or conditions raise the levels of these endorphins in the brain, what lowers them, and how painful disorders or helpful therapies affect the endorphin system are but a few of the important questions that scientific research is currently attempting to answer. Acupuncture may, for example, temporarily diminish sensations of pain by causing an elevation of the endorphin level.

These and future breakthroughs will ultimately lead to a better understanding of the mysteries of pain and the drugs used to treat it.

Mood-Altering Drugs—The successful alleviation of pain, including headache pain, cannot always be achieved with analgesics. Emotions, such as anxiety and depression, influence the feeling of pain and its meaning to those suffering from it.

Two types of mood-altering medications are used in treating

pain: medications that reduce anxiety and tension, and medications that raise spirits. The anxiety reducers are called tranquilizers, and the latter are called antidepressants.

TRANQUILIZERS: There are two types of tranquilizers. The minor tranquilizers are used for treating mild to moderate degrees of anxiety and tension. The major tranquilizers are used to treat severe states of agitation and to modify the abnormal behavior often associated with serious emotional disorders. Included in the group of minor tranquilizers are chlorazapate (Tranxene), chlordiazepoxide (Librium), diazepam (Valium), meprobamate (Miltown and Equanil), and phenobarbitol.

Like all drugs, tranquilizers have the potential for producing side effects, sometimes serious ones, even when taken in recommended dosages. Low dosages of mild tranquilizers may cause drowsiness and a loss of coordination that resembles drunkenness. These reactions tend to occur when the patient first begins taking the medication, but can develop later when an accumulation of the medication occurs. Prolonged use of the minor tranquilizers can result in dependence on them. Sudden reduction of high doses of these drugs can cause withdrawal reactions, including epileptic-like seizures.

A significant depression of mood can be a side effect of prolonged use of tranquilizers. Occasionally this results in a depressed, tearful, and uninterested state. Some people taking standard doses of tranquilizing medications report that they are unable to refrain from weeping over even small problems or frustrations. An overdose of tranquilizers, such as in suicide attempts, causes serious impairment of brain function, coma, cessation of breathing, and even death. Taking tranquilizers in combination with alcohol enhances the danger of fatal toxicity, even if they are taken several hours apart.

The major tranquilizers, such as chlorpromazine (Thorazine), prochlorperazine (Compazine), and perphenazine (Trilafon), used formerly for only severe psychiatric states such as schizophrenia, have also recently been used with success in the treatment of chronic pain. While these tranquilizers are not as "addicting" as the minor tranquilizers, they carry with their use a significantly greater medical risk. Nonetheless, current research as well as clini-

Table II Sinus Headache Remedies

Name	Active Ingredients/Tablet	Effect
Sine-Off	325 mg. Aspirin 2 mg. Chlorpheniramine maleate 18.75 mg. Phenylpropanolamine	Analgesic Antihistamine Decongestant (vasoconstrictor)
Sine-Aid	325 mg. Acetaminophen 25 mg. Phenylpropanolamine	Analgesic Decongestant (vasoconstrictor)
Sinarest	325 mg. Acetaminophen 2 mg. Chlorpheniramine maleate 18.75 mg. Phenylpropanolamine	Analgesic Antihistamine Decongestant (vasoconstrictor)
Sinutab	325 mg. Acetaminophen 25 mg. Phenylpropanolamine 22 mg. Phenyltoloxamine	Analgesic Decongestant (vasoconstrictor) Antihistamine
Dristan	325 mg. Aspirin 5 mg. Phenylephrine 2 mg. Chlorpheniramine maleate 16.2 mg. Caffeine	Analgesic Decongestant (vasoconstrictor) Antihistamine See text

cal experience suggest that the major tranquilizers may mitigate chronic pain through different mechanisms than those used for tranquilization.

For a variety of biological and psychological reasons, tranquilizers are frequently abused; this should discourage their casual use. When employed cautiously and for limited periods of time, however, tranquilizers may be occasionally helpful in treating some forms of head pain.

Minor tranqualizers are not particularly useful for stopping an exsiting headache, although they may assist in sedating the victim during the discomfort and sometimes are used to control the

Comment

Can raise blood pressure with
sustained use of high dosages

Can raise blood pressure with
sustained use of high dosages

Can raise blood pressure with
sustained use of high dosages

Can raise blood pressure with
sustained use of high dosages
Sedating

Can raise blood pressure and
affect heart rate with sustained use of high dosages
Unreliable absorption from
stomach (decongestant)
Sedating

---

anxiety that can trigger a headache. The major tranquilizers (see
above) may be used in some instances to reverse an existing headache, as well as to control the nausea that often accompanies
migraine.

During the past several years, there has been a growing concern
about the indiscriminate use of tranquilizers, because of the many
problems that have resulted from such widespread and often
inappropriate use. While the authors of this book agree that these
drugs do not necessarily have a place in the treatment of all patients experiencing stress or who have anxious moments in their
life, it is likewise important to recognize that stress is a major

health hazard. It is impossible to measure the negative influence of stress in our society, but many physicians believe that stress, through biological mechanisms, enhances the risk of serious illness, ranging from heart attack to cancer. While we are not suggesting that the use of minor tranquilizers may indeed alter these consequences, it must be said that if a patient benefits from appropriate doses and limited usage of a tranquilizer, then perhaps the patient should not be made to feel guilty or inferior. Not everyone can afford long-term psychotherapy to help alleviate stress or anxiety. While effective nonmedicinal intervention is *always* desirable, the temporary use of tranquilizing medication may be, at times, the compromise of choice. Patients need to be carefully instructed in the use of these medications in the proper way for specific reasons, and within an agreed upon time limit. Open and trusting communication between you and your doctor regarding the use of these medications, their limitations, and their hazards is essential.

ANTIDEPRESSANTS: Depression can be a serious and disabling condition that can vary greatly in its intensity and disruptive influence. Being depressed, in the medical sense, is not just feeling "blue" or being "down." Nor is depression simply the temporary sadness that follows tragic or disappointing experiences. Depression is an abnormal mental state that can have a devastating impact upon one's ability to function. Depression can cause a slowing of mental and physical activity, keeping patients in bed and making all contact difficult for days or weeks at a time. Some people who suffer depression are not slowed but are anxiously restless, a condition known as agitated depression. This condition is often confused with anxiety.

The following is a passage from a letter that a patient wrote because of her "nerves." It demonstrates the smothering effect of her depression.

... I am regressing again. I've been regressing since Friday. I think I could make it if I could just find someone to talk to when I'm regressing.

I've been drunk all weekend. I shouldn't mix pills and beer, but who cares!

These regressions are the awfulest things. You feel like you are in a world of your own and nobody can reach you and you can't reach anybody else. It reminds me of a swimmer trying to get to the top so they can get air but they never make it . . .

(This patient was placed in the care of a psychiatrist and she is now considerably improved.)

Attempts at suicide are not uncommon during periods of depression. Suicide is most likely when the depression begins to improve, since in depression's deepest phases the slowing of mental processes and the reduction of activity are somewhat protective against an aggressive acting out against oneself.

Depression often accompanies recurring headaches. It is difficult to determine whether the depression helps cause the headaches or occurs as a result of the chronic pain. Numerous research studies, however, clearly show that at least 50 percent of people with daily or almost daily headaches also possess elements of depression. Dr. Seymour Diamond of Chicago, a noted headache authority, recognized this and coined the term "depression headache" for some headache conditions. Treating depression is an important part of the total treatment of many chronic headache problems.

Antidepressants are beneficial for some types of depression because they increase the amount of some brain chemicals. Lower than normal quantities of these substances are present in some depressed individuals. There are two types of antidepressants: the tricyclic group, a term referring to this group's chemical structure, and the monoamine oxidase (MAO) inhibitors, a term reflecting the medication's method of action. The tricyclics are the type most often used in pain therapy.

Among the frequently used tricyclic antidepressants are amitriptyline (Elavil and Endep), doxepin (Sinequan), imipramine (Tofranil), and nortriptyline (Aventyl and Pamelor). There are many others. Adverse effects of the tricyclics include a dry mouth, drowsiness, blurred vision, tingling fingers, and occasionally changes in blood pressure, heart rhythm, and pulse rate. Two additional complications associated with tricyclic antidepressant therapy are changes in behavior and a sometimes uncontrollable twitching or jerking movement of the face or the arms and legs. However, most people taking these antidepressants do not experience serious side reactions.

Antidepressants, like the tranquilizers mentioned in the previous section, are capable of stimulating appetite and also causing a change in the way the body metabolizes food. As a result, many patients taking these drugs, while enjoying a less painful existence, may find themselves gaining weight unexpectedly. Sometimes this weight gain is associated with an increase of appetite, either stimulated by the medicines or from a state of well-being because of the relief of pain. This unwanted side effect, while not serious in itself, can usually be overcome by careful monitoring of calories and an aggressive exercise program, both of which represent good health practices anyway.

The tricyclic antidepressants and perhaps the MAO inhibitors as well may be effective in treating headache in a way not directly related to their use in the relief of depression. These drugs may work by raising the pain threshold. Much more research on this issue is needed to understand this complex problem.

The MAO inhibitor antidepressants block (inhibit) an important enzyme called monoamine oxidase, which reduces the level of some of the brain chemicals. By blocking this enzyme, the level of certain chemicals is thought to remain at a higher level.

The most serious problem associated with the use of the monoamine oxidase inhibitor antidepressants is the need to avoid foods and drinks that contain the chemical tyramine. Ingestion of tyramine or related substances, while at the same time blocking the body's ability to metabolize them, can result in a dangerous elevation of blood pressure, among other symptoms. Among the foods that must be restricted when taking the monoamine oxidase inhibitors are Chianti, sherry, and several other wines, chocolates, beer, aged cheese, sour cream, nuts, soy sauce, and yeast extracts. If you take these enzyme-inhibiting drugs, your physician must provide you with a complete list of foods to avoid.

When antidepressants are used in headache therapy, they are always used preventively since they have no value once the headache has developed.

Treating Headache with Specialized Drugs—In many headache situations, mood-altering medications and analgesics are either inappropriate or ineffective and these situations require specialized drugs. These specialized drugs do not actually affect the ability to feel pain, as do analgesics, but instead counteract the abnormality considered responsible for the development of the headache.

In migraine, for example, there is vasodilation, an abnormal widening of blood vessel diameter. Drugs that constrict these dilated blood vessels often relieve the migraine headache, although the reason for their effectiveness may not be confined to vasoconstriction alone. The vasoconstrictors most often used in the treatment of migraine are prepared from the plant fungus called ergot. This fungus grows on a number of grains, particularly rye. Many drugs are derived from ergot, and the form most frequently used for the treatment of migraine is called ergotamine tartrate. Ergotamine tartrate can be prepared to be taken by a variety of routes: oral, rectal, subcutaneous, sublingual (under the tongue), or by inhalation.

Among the complications associated with ergot overdosage are hallucinations and seizures. Severe constriction of blood vessels throughout the body may also occur when too much ergot is taken. A report in *Science* magazine* suggests that the bizarre behavior attributed to witchcraft in Salem, Massachusetts, may have resulted from ergot poisoning due to contaminated rye. The drug LSD (lysergic acid diethylamide) is chemically related to ergot.

The ergot-containing drugs are most often used to stop, or abort, rather than prevent, a migraine headache. A more detailed discussion of these medications will be found in Chapter 2.

Methysergide (Sansert) is another specific antimigraine medication, but it is used in the preventive approach rather than the abortive approach. It has little value once a headache has begun. It, like ergot, is chemically related to LSD.

Another drug currently being used in migraine prevention was initially used for heart patients suffering from coronary artery disease. This drug, called propranolol (Inderal), was found quite by accident to prevent migraine attacks in some of the heart patients who also suffered from migraine. Both Sansert and Inderal will be discussed in Chapter 2 along with other medications used to treat migraine.

Another specific type of medication used in certain types of headaches are the muscle relaxants, often used in combination with other drugs to treat the headache produced by muscle con-

* L. R. Caporael, "The Satan Loosed in Salem?" *Science* (April 2, 1976), p. 192.

traction. The muscle contraction headache is frequently called the tension headache, and much of the pain in this disorder results from contraction of the muscles of the neck, scalp, and face. Drugs that relieve these muscle spasms may help alleviate the tightening tension and control pain.

Many more drugs useful for treating headache will be discussed in the appropriate sections of the chapters covering the specific headache conditions.

TREATING HEADACHE WITHOUT DRUGS

Although drugs have represented the mainstay of traditional headache treatments, it is important to try to find safer and equally effective means of relieving or preventing headaches without resorting to the use of drugs. Because emotional factors play an important role in the genesis of many headaches, any method of headache treatment that relieves stress, anxiety, or depression can be helpful in preventing some headaches. Literally defined, psychotherapy means treating the mind, but in the broad sense, it can include any method of lessening tension, anxiety, and depression. Psychotherapy, in this sense, ranges from an informal discussion with a friend or marriage partner to a formal professional interaction between a psychologist or psychiatrist and a patient.

Simple therapies may help to relieve headache pain or prevent headache completely. Heat applied to the back of the neck, cold packs around the head, or massage of sore neck and temple muscles may be beneficial for some headaches. Those suffering from muscle contraction headaches, particularly, benefit from an improvement in posture, wearing a supportive neck collar, using a simple device offering gentle neck traction, or improvement of dental or jaw problems if they exist.

Currently, there is increasing interest in the potential value of relaxation techniques. The methods of relaxing vary from simple and informal relaxation exercises to control overtense muscles to more structured and formally taught mind-control techniques. Regular exercise, reading, hobbies, or sipping a soothing beverage are all familiar methods of relaxing and can be important in achieving a feeling of calm. Alcoholic beverages and other intoxicants are used for relaxation by many people, but the potential for abuse prevents us from advocating this form of therapy for headache problems. Alcohol may actually relieve a muscle contraction headache, but it can trigger a cluster headache or a migraine headache.

The formal relaxation methods include meditation, yoga, and biofeedback. Meditation is a means of achieving relaxation by the repetition of specially chosen words during two twenty-minute sessions each day. Meditations may afford both biological as well as emotional benefits for those who practice the technique regularly, although the therapeutic impact of meditation is not yet fully understood.

Biofeedback training is a means of teaching you to develop a conscious control over various automatic body functions. The tightness of your neck muscles or even the temperature of your fingers can be altered through control over your body. A variety of devices can be used to help you achieve this control, and the proponents of biofeedback training assert that many disorders, including muscle contraction headaches and migraine headaches, can be relieved with the regular use of biofeedback. Evidence is rapidly accumulating that biofeedback, when taught by competent professionals and used regularly by the patient, may have an impressive impact on many headache sufferers. We advocate its use for selected headache patients. It is our opinion, however, that biofeedback itself should be only a *component* of a broader therapy program. What appears most important is the scope of the program in which behavior, expression of anger, identification of stress-producing mechanisms, and other related issues are confronted. Simply being put into a room with a machine and being told to "do it yourself" is, in our opinion, an inappropriate way to administer the therapy. When used in conjunction with other therapeutic techniques, biofeedback can be helpful with some patients. Recently the American Association for the Study of Headaches recommended biofeedback as an effective method of treating headaches in appropriate cases.

Acupuncture continues to be a controversial form of therapy, and the many unsubstantiated claims of cures must be greeted with skepticism. Acupuncture is the insertion of special needles into specific predetermined areas of the body. Many of these acupuncture locations have been determined by ancient Chinese medical teachings. There are many theories that attempt to explain how acupuncture relieves pain in some individuals, and final judgment regarding acupuncture's effectiveness must be reserved until well-controlled studies convincingly demonstrate its benefit beyond the placebo response. As mentioned earlier, *preliminary* data suggest that acupuncture's temporary effect *may* be related to increased levels of endorphins.

Biofeedback and acupuncture seem innocent since they do not carry with them detrimental side effects. But consumer naiveté, together with premature and unsubstantiated claims, has created a good deal of exploitation in the field of headache cures. Objective scientific investigation must be carried out before reliable conclusions can be made. It should be of great concern that these new and "revolutionary" therapies are sometimes performed by practitioners who are unqualified. Generally, we advise against using any method except under the supervision of qualified professional personnel.

Many of our headache patients who are joggers suggest that a headache can be aborted by jogging. Some even suggest that they have suffered far fewer headaches since taking up a regular exercise program. Some psychiatrists and psychologists believe that exercise such as this may also play a beneficial role in the treatment of anxiety and depression, as well as other emotional problems. These possible benefits could represent merely placebo responses, and a firm conclusion must await more scientifically designed means of evaluation. However, it is our belief that regular exercise such as jogging, lasting 15 to 20 minutes a day, four times a week, for patients whose doctors say they are physically fit, *may* be helpful to both mind and body.

The discussion of treatment must address the subject of chiropractic therapies because many people with headaches have tried these in their desperate search for relief of painful symptoms. As neurologists, we feel that we have a responsibility to offer you an opinion on this subject, because the basic theory of the chiropractic approach is that all or most diseases arise because of compression on nerve structures.

We do not believe that chiropractic theory and practice have any convincing basis in modern scientific knowledge. It appears to us that chiropractors ignore the scientific evidence accumulated during years of legitimate medical research. In our opinion, they are not adequately trained to diagnose or treat many of the medical disorders for which often desperate patients seek their help.

The chiropractic theory is based on a belief that disease is due to a displacement (subluxation) of vertebrae. This, chiropractors claim, results in abnormalities of nerve function. Diseases are a consequence. We know of no scientific evidence suggesting that cancer, heart disease, lung disease, or most other disease entities, including most cases of pain about the head, have any convincing or consistent relationship to displaced vertebrae or compressed nerves. With rare exceptions, the X rays of patients diagnosed by chiropractors as showing displaced vertebrae as the cause of their symptoms have, upon review, failed to reveal significant abnormalities.

Chiropractors frequently show patients their X rays, suggesting that certain bones of the spinal column are misaligned. In fact, patients frequently report that they could see that the vertebrae were not in perfect alignment. However, the backbones are *not* normally in perfect alignment. The curvature of the spine is nature's way of giving adequate flexibility and support to the vertebral column. One clear example is the "bump" that you can feel in the lower center of your neck. This bump is actually a part of the seventh neck (cervical) vertebra, which is normally "displaced" backwards a few millimeters. This is the *normal* position for this vertebra. On X ray, the untrained eye would consider this vertebra misaligned or subluxated. Furthermore, the relative position of the vertebrae may change as the position of the head and neck change. In essence, this means that a highly skilled professional is required to accurately interpret X rays in order to determine whether the vertebrae are truly in proper location. Subluxation of vertebrae is a *rare* phenomenon in medical practice, and if present can pose a serious medical risk. We believe that physicians, such as radiologists, whose careers and training are focused upon interpretation of X-ray abnormalities, are required for accurate assessment of these conditions.

Chiropractors perform their therapeutic intervention by manipulating the spine. A concern of many medical doctors is the potential hazard incurred by this manipulative technique. The spinal cord runs down the center of the backbone and its delicate nerves emerge from between the vertebrae. The spinal cord itself has approximately the same circumference as a carrot, and is extraordinarily fragile. Nature designed the back to be rigid in order to protect fragile nerve tissue from damage that can be expected from excessive movement of the vertebrae. The back muscles participate in the support as do the tendons, which are designed to hold the vertebrae in close approximation. Any effort, beyond simple exercise, massage, or traction, that stretches, twists, or otherwise unnaturally imposes strain on this important system must in our opinion be considered potentially hazardous.

Additionally, it is our opinion that chiropractors are not trained to diagnose the many medical symptoms for which people often seek their help. It is of great concern to us that any delay in establishing an accurate diagnosis of serious and possibly life-threatening conditions for even a few weeks can prove fatal.

Finally, we recognize that many patients, particularly those with muscle spasm as part of their headache problem, do benefit from any measure that relieves spasm; a firm, gentle massage of neck muscles or traction will do this. But chiropractic treatment frequently goes beyond this, and we cannot recommend it.*

This chapter ends by suggesting that the most useful therapeutic tool that any physician can possess is the trust and respect of the patient. But you are cautioned against bestowing this respect simply because your physician is called "doctor." Your trust and respect must be earned, not only through competence but also by the manner in which your physician relates to you. Your doctor must be willing to try to relieve your discomfort by the most effective and safest means possible. For your part, you must recognize that human illnesses, particularly pain, are very difficult to treat, and trying to do so safely is a time-consuming and sometimes frustrating challenge. If your doctor is committed to helping you and does so in a medically qualified way, you must be as patient with your physician as he or she must be with you. Patience, trust, and respect must be mutually earned and extended.

* For an excellent, objective two-part review of chiropractic, see *Consumer Reports*, September 1975, page 542, and October 1975, page 606.

Chapter 2 Migraine Headaches

THE MIGRAINE PROFILE

The Migraine Profile below is a description of the symptoms of a migraine. It is followed by a series of questions that a physician might ask you if migraine were suspected as the diagnosis.

Warning: This exercise is not a means of diagnosing your headaches. The exercise is provided only to encourage you to carefully consider the features of your own headaches using a characterization of migraine for comparison. An accurate diagnosis of your headache problem requires a thorough medical evaluation by a trained professional. There is no acceptable substitute.

Profile

Although you feel well between attacks, you have headaches that occur in distinct episodes of discomfort. The headache can last from hours to days. You are likely to experience nausea and maybe vomiting, and a sick feeling throughout your body during the headaches is common. This is particularly true during the more intense attacks. When the attack is over, you may feel "washed out" for days.

Your attacks may be preceded or accompanied by symptoms that may include light sensitivity and flashing, glaring, or glittering lights in your vision. You may experience partial loss of vision. The attacks may be preceded by weakness or numbness on one side of your body, double vision, or difficulty in speaking correctly.

Your headaches can occur without a warning except perhaps a vague sick feeling a day or so before the attack. You may have noticed that this feeling often heralds an attack.

It is likely that your head hurts more on one side than the other. The pain may settle around your forehead, the top of your head, or behind, over, or in one or both eyes or temples. Your headaches are frequent, but not necessarily, throbbing, pounding, or boring. Sometimes your neck as well as your head aches.

Your headaches can actually awaken you from sleep, and they may begin at any time of the day. Certain foods, weather changes, stress, menstrual periods, or alcoholic beverages may trigger or worsen an attack. Bending over during an attack may intensify the pain. Other members of your family may have similar headaches.

If this general description of a migraine is similar to your headaches, you may want to answer the following questions. The questions are typical of some of those that would be asked of you if your physician suspected a diagnosis of migraine.

	True	False
1. There is a history of similar headaches in your family.	——	——
2. Assuming you are an adult, your headaches began in childhood, adolescence, or early twenties.	——	——
3. As a child you experienced frequent and unexplained nausea and vomiting or abdominal pain, particularly when you were excited or looking forward to an unusual event.	——	——
4. You were prone to motion sickness as a child.	——	——

True   False

5. Your headaches sometimes wake you up in the middle of the night. ___ ___

6. Your headaches can be brought on or aggravated by drinking alcohol. ___ ___

7. Your headaches tend to throb or pound. ___ ___

8. Between your attacks, you are in otherwise normal health. ___ ___

9. During a headache, your eyes become very sensitive to light. ___ ___

10. Sounds become irritating to you during your headaches. ___ ___

11. You seek a dark, quiet room during your headaches rather than preoccupying yourself with activity. ___ ___

12. Bending over makes your headaches worse. ___ ___

13. Your headaches frequently occur during your menstrual cycle or a day or two before or after it. ___ ___

14. You have nausea and vomiting with your headaches. ___ ___

15. Your headaches often occur on weekends, holidays, vacations, or during a "letdown" period after great stress or excitement. ___ ___

16. Your headaches seem to be triggered by going without eating for six hours or more. ___ ___

17. Certain foods and beverages, such as wine, cheese, chocolate, vanilla, citrus fruits, hot dogs, fatty foods, yogurt, and soy sauce, trigger or worsen your headaches. ___ ___

18. After your attacks, you are exhausted for hours or days. ___ ___

The characterization that you have just read and the questions that have been asked represent a profile of the migraine syndrome. If your headaches are similar to this presentation, please read carefully the following discussion about migraine.

THE MIGRAINE

A migraine is not simply any bad headache. Although an ache or pain in the head is the most characteristic feature of most migraine attacks, many individuals experience only minor discomfort and a few have no actual pain at all. A migraine attack may be a severe headache on one occasion and no more than an annoying discomfort, located elsewhere around the head or face, on another. Migraine is an intriguing disorder, and despite its having been recognized for centuries and having affected millions upon millions of people, this baffling condition continues to defy a clear understanding of its cause.

The term "migraine" is of French origin, but was derived from a Greek term meaning an affliction of half of the head (hemicrania). An old English term was "megrim."

Migraine's numerous symptoms reflect involvement of many parts of the body, including the gastrointestinal tract and the eyes. Frequently the symptoms of a migraine attack mimic those of strokes, brain tumors, and epilepsy.

A syndrome is defined as a group of symptoms often occurring together and resulting from a basic abnormal condition. Migraine is considered a syndrome. In a syndrome like migraine, the symptoms may develop all at one time or be staggered in their onset during the course of the illness.

Migraine belongs to the group of conditions referred to as vascular headaches. In this group are various other painful syndromes affecting the face and head. In addition to pain, a common feature of all these disorders is an abnormal fluctuation in the size of blood vessels in the head, face, and neck, as well as other parts of the body.

THE CAUSE OF THE MIGRAINE SYNDROME

In spite of years of research, the exact cause of migraine remains unknown. Excessive widening of some blood vessels and narrowing, or constricting, of others play an important role in producing the pain and other unpleasant sensations associated with migraine.

Enlarging (dilation) of the blood vessels of the scalp and face causes pain by exerting pressure on nerves that lie in or around the affected arteries and veins. Narrowing of other blood vessels leads to a diminished supply of blood to various parts of the brain, and this can result in an impairment of brain function. The malfunctioning of these brain areas is reflected by the temporary neurological symptoms associated with many migraine attacks, such as numbness, weakness, or visual impairment. In persons predisposed to migraine, both biological and emotional factors can trigger this abnormal reaction of blood vessels.

Current evidence suggests that the blood vessels of individuals with migraine may simply overreact to a variety of normal stimuli, much like blushing easily when embarrassed or turning pale suddenly when frightened.

Abnormalities of blood vessel size, however, represent only part of the problem in migraine. An inflammation of the tissue around the blood vessels and the accumulation of chemical irritants in the region of the affected veins and arteries have also been detected through scientific research. One of these substances is called neurokinin and is similar to a chemical present in wasp venom.

Much of the current research on migraine focuses on a chemical substance called serotonin. Serotonin is found in a variety of tissues, including the brain, and is suspected of playing a key role in the production of the migraine syndrome. Serotonin constricts some blood vessels and dilates others.

Serotonin is a nitrogen-containing substance called an amine. Like other brain amines, such as noradrenaline, it has an important influence in determining the size of blood vessels, mood, and even sleep patterns. Very low levels of these amines, for example, may be responsible for severe depression, whereas an overabundance may result in the opposite mood, mania.

The level of serotonin in the blood drops dramatically as the migraine attack begins, and a number of medications used to control migraine have a chemical formula similar to serotonin and may substitute for serotonin when levels of it fall.

Other important chemicals of current interest are substances called prostaglandins. Prostaglandins were first thought to come from the male prostate gland but are now recognized to be present in many organs of both men and women. There are many different types of prostaglandins, and research has shown that some of them when injected into volunteers who were not migraine sufferers produced symptoms very close to those of a migraine headache.*

Recently, interest has focused on blood-platelet abnormalities in migraine. The platelets are important components of the clotting mechanism, and current research has shown them to be abnormal in migraine patients.

In summary, migraine is considered a condition in which a number of biological reactions may occur throughout the entire body. The tendency for "overreactivity" may be biologically predetermined or "programmed." Once present, this biological programming may be influenced by a variety of physiological as well as emotional triggering events that will determine the frequency, nature, and severity of the headache attack. Some authorities believe that the migraine potential represents an overactive "protective" response, in which various organ systems respond to what is perceived as a threat, either physiological or emotional. Ironically, the protective response may be more uncomfortable than the perceived threat.

THE TWO TYPES OF MIGRAINE

Migraine is divided into two major forms, the classical migraine and the common migraine. The common variety accounts for approximately 80 percent of all migraine attacks, although ironically it is the less frequently occurring classical form that is the most familiar and the easiest to diagnose. The term "classical" is applied because of the many historical references to this form of the syndrome.

Migraine is divided into these two types because differences exist between their symptom patterns, although both do share the common feature of headache and are thought to come from the same or similar biological abnormalities. In many people, attacks share features of both types of migraine and a separation into distinct forms is impossible.

* L. A. Carlsson, L. G. Ekelund, and L. Oro, "Clinical and Metabolic Effects of Different Doses of Prostaglandins on Man," in *Acta Medica Scandinavica* (May 1968), p. 183.

SYMPTOMS OF CLASSICAL MIGRAINE

In classical migraine the attack occurs in two phases. The first phase begins before the headache develops and is appropriately called the preheadache phase, or the prodrome. The word "prodrome" comes from the Greek word *"prodromos,"* meaning running (*dromos*) before (*pro*). The preheadache phase usually begins approximately ten to thirty minutes before the beginning of the headache phase and is characterized by one or more of several symptoms.

Visual symptoms represent the most common preheadache disturbance in the classical migraine, varying from blurriness to partial blindness. The visual symptoms are often dramatic (see Photos A–F). Some people describe "flashbulb" blind spots occurring in one or, more commonly, both eyes. Others have the experience of illuminating or sparkling phenomena appearing as either small spots or unusual shapes and forms. Some of these phenomena are multicolored as well. One common pattern is called the "fortification spectra," an elaborately designed zigzag form that glares or scintillates like a neon sign. The fortification spectra gets its name from the complex zigzag walls that were constructed around embattled cities for fortification.

During the preheadache phase, a partial blindness may occur. This blindness may take the form of a decrease or a complete loss of vision in one-half of each eye, a condition known as hemianopsia. An irregular blind spot located somewhere in the field of vision is also a common preheadache symptom. This blind area is called a scotoma. It is an island, or spot, of decreased or absent vision within an otherwise normal visual field. A person with a scotoma may, when peering into a mirror, be unable to see his/her own nose, ear, face, or other area, depending upon the scotoma's size and location.

Occasionally migraine victims report tunnel vision, an effect that is like looking through binoculars. Some patients bump into or stumble over objects during the preheadache phase of their attacks, citing clumsiness as the reason, when impairment of their side, or peripheral, vision is actually to blame.

Another bizarre visual phenomenon that can occur in migraine during the preheadache phase is referred to as the Alice in Wonderland syndrome. Lewis Carroll suffered from classical migraine. It is possible that many of the unusual events depicted in Alice's adventures actually reflect some of Lewis Carroll's own migraine patterns, such as alterations in shape, hearing, taste, smell, touch, and body image. Photographs E and F demonstrate the bizarre visual hallucinations that, along with distortions of smell and taste, are referred to as the Alice in Wonderland syndrome when present in patients with migraine. Photograph F is an actual page from *Alice's Adventures in Wonderland*, illustrated by John Tenniel with the assistance of Lewis Carroll.*

While visual impairment is perhaps the most common preheadache symptom and may represent the only preheadache complaint, other dramatic nonvisual disturbances can also occur. A temporary weakness and sensory symptoms similar to numbness or tingling may develop on one side of the body or one section of the body. Slurring of words or an inability to express one's self clearly may develop. Some victims experience increased sensitivity of their skin, which causes irritation when the skin is lightly touched.

Other symptoms that may occur in the preheadache phase include mental confusion, irritability, unexpected exhaustion and fatigue, mild fever, flushing or pallor, sweating, and dizziness. Some individuals describe a swelling in various parts of their body, while others state that they have diarrhea or an increased need to urinate. The hands and feet may become cold. Abdominal pain may also occur during the preheadache phase, although "abdominal migraine" is more common in children than in adults.

Many of the preheadache symptoms, particularly the ones related to neurological disturbances, such as weakness, visual distortions, and numbness or tingling, are believed to result from impaired blood circulation to specific areas of the brain. When these symptoms begin suddenly, they may seem like the beginning of a stroke. The neurological abnormalities may remain for some

---

* See end of chapter for more on the Alice in Wonderland syndrome.

time after the preheadache period ends and, rarely, they become permanent disabilities.

Depending on one's imagination, it is possible to find many references in Alice's adventures that suggest symptoms of migraine. For example, the following is found in *Through the Looking Glass:*

> The sun was shining on the sea
>   Shining with all his might:
> He did his very best to make
>   The billows smooth and bright—
> And this was odd, because it was
>   The middle of the night.
>
> The moon was shining sulkily,
>   Because she thought the sun
> Had got no business to be there
>   After the day was done—
> 'It's very rude of him,' she said
>   'To come and spoil the fun!'

Is the sea, shining with all his might, a reference to the scintillating light phenomena that accompany so many migraine attacks? " 'It's very rude of him,' she said, 'To come and spoil the fun!' " Could this statement refer to the disruptive influence that a migraine headache can have?

The following passage is from the chapter "Queen Alice":

> "Take care of yourself!" screamed the White Queen, seizing Alice's hair with both her hands. "Something's going to happen!"
> And then (as Alice afterwards described it) all sorts of things happened in a moment. The candles all grew up to the ceiling, looking something like a bed of rushes with fireworks at the top. As to the bottles, they each took a pair of plates, which they hastily fitted on as wings, and so, with forks for legs, went fluttering about in all directions: "and very like birds they look," . . .

Notice the references to abnormal shapes and sizes, flickering lights, and the head, the latter suggested by the White Queen seizing Alice's hair with both hands.

THE HEADACHE PHASE OF CLASSICAL MIGRAINE

Usually within fifteen to twenty minutes after the preheadache symptoms begin, they diminish. It is at about this time that the headache develops. At first the headache may be mild, but it gradually worsens. The pain may initially be felt on only one side, but as it intensifies, it may spread to involve most of the head. The pain can develop on both sides simultaneously, and the scalp, face, and neck may be tender to touch. The ache is frequently dull, deep, and throbbing, and often begins in the forehead, ear, jaw, or in or around an eye or temple.

Shoulder and neck pain may develop. In part this is due to muscle spasm resulting automatically from the pain around the neck and head or as part of an attempt to hold the painful head motionless, since migraine pain is frequently worsened by head movement, bending over, sneezing, or coughing. It is not unusual, understandably, for a muscle-spasm-type headache to be superimposed on the migraine.

Nausea, vomiting, mental cloudiness, total body achiness, abdominal pain, chills, and cold hands and feet commonly accompany the headache.

The actual attack of classical migraine usually lasts from one hour to more than a day. Following it, sore muscles, total body exhaustion, and a continued mild mental cloudiness may persist for days.

These attacks do not all follow the same pattern. Occasionally, the headache of the classical migraine variety is mild in intensity and not particularly debilitating. If the pain is either mild or absent and is not mentioned to the physician, it may become very difficult to establish a correct diagnosis. In rare cases, the headache phase precedes the other symptoms in classical migraine. The following example illustrates the difficulty in diagnosing a classical migraine when the features of an attack vary from the usual:

A 22-year-old student at a nearby university experienced recurring episodes of "I can't understand what I am reading." These attacks usually occurred after he had been concentrating for several hours, especially on biophysics problems. Without warning, he would realize that he could no longer see the letters and numbers in the papers and book, but he could see images on either side of them. His central field of vision was blurred and out of focus. A year before, when these attacks first began, he had studied his face in a mirror to see if anything was wrong with his eyes. To his great concern, he could see his ears and cheeks but not his eyes or nose. He attributed this visual impairment to eyestrain and made a practice of going to sleep soon after the onset of each episode. Upon awakening, he ordinarily felt "perfectly okay."

On the day I was called to the emergency room to examine this patient, he had experienced another episode of visual impairment, but instead of going to sleep as was customary, he decided to attend a lecture. About one hour after the onset of the visual difficulties, the patient developed a severe pain in his right eye. According to the patient, this was the first time that pain had occurred.

Aspirin did not help to alleviate the pain and he concluded that the severe pain resulted from "an insufficient supply of blood to my brain." Treating himself, he tried to remedy this deficient blood supply by placing his head lower than the rest of the body to "increase the brain's blood supply." This maneuver only intensified the pain, but he realized that his visual impairment was no longer present. Soon he fell asleep, and on awakening he had only a mild headache. Although the headache had passed, he was very concerned and decided to go to the hospital for treatment.

When he was first questioned about experiencing a headache in connection with the visual episodes, the answer was no. But later, he remembered that on a few occasions, when he had not fallen asleep immediately after the beginning of the visual problems, he had developed a mild and not particularly bothersome discomfort around the eyes.

The diagnosis in this patient was classical migraine, and this case demonstrated two problems in establishing a diagnosis. The first was the practice of falling asleep soon after the onset of visual disturbances so that the victim was actually unaware of the headache phase of his attacks. Secondly, the patient's initial description of his visual symptoms reflected the mistaken belief that he was having a problem with his ability to understand the material he was studying rather than impairment of vision being responsible for his inability to read.

The current research in migraine headache suggests that individuals with frequent attacks of classical migraine, particularly those headaches associated with significant neurological symptoms, *may* be more likely than the nonmigraine person to suffer from strokes and heart attacks later in life. This tendency may be related to an abnormality of the blood particles called platelets that play an important role in the normal clotting process. An increase of platelet stickiness or other abnormalities of the platelets can account for this clotting tendency, and current research is looking into the possibility that treating classical migraine sufferers with medications that decrease the platelet stickiness may improve the long-term health of migraine patients. Plain aspirin is one such medication.

SYMPTOMS OF COMMON MIGRAINE

The most common form of migraine headache is appropriately called the common migraine. Unlike the classical type, the common migraine headache does not have distinctive phases. However, many of our patients report that hours or even days prior to an attack they experience various nonspecific symptoms, including mental cloudiness, unexpected mood changes, a noticeable gain in weight, and general fatigue. Some patients can reliably predict the onset of a headache as a result of these heralding symptoms.

Some people state that just prior to an attack an overall sick feeling and irritability occur. One person told us that she becomes a "real bitch" the day before a migraine attack. Many patients tell us that they experience an intense craving for chocolate or salt prior to the onset of a headache.

Every so often an individual with migraine will experience a swelling of various parts of the body prior to the onset of the headache. This swelling is called edema (oedema), a word of Greek origin meaning an accumulation of fluid that results in swelling.

In addition to its lack of clear-cut phases, another feature distinguishing the common migraine from the classical migraine is that it is not unusual for common migraine to persist for at least three or four days before it subsides. The headache itself is quite similar to that of classical migraine except that the pain more frequently spreads throughout the head, face, and jaw, and occasionally localizes in the back of the head and in the neck region. The headache may be more intense on one side of the head and face, but the emphasis can shift from side to side in alternate attacks. This shifting of the painful area can also be a symptom of many classical migraine episodes.

Migraine headaches can awaken their victim from sleep during the night or early-morning hours. Nocturnal awakening with pain is a feature common to vascular headaches (migraine and cluster headaches) and is rarely seen in other types of headache conditions. Awakening in the morning with a headache, however, is common to many different types of headaches.

It is unusual for clear-cut neurological symptoms to occur in common migraine, but nausea and vomiting, diarrhea, and increased urination are very common during the three- or four-day ordeal. Some victims who vomit and cannot eat or drink during their attacks may lose enough fluid from their systems to become dehydrated. An increased sensitivity to odors is not unusual during an attack and may help bring on some of the nausea and vomiting, but other explanations, such as the presence of circulating chemical substances in the victim's blood during migraine attacks, may also play a role in producing the nausea and vomiting.

Sensitivity to light, called photophobia, and increased sensitivity to sound, known as hyperacusis, frequently accompany the nausea and vomiting in the common migraine attack. They can also be evident in the classical form of migraine. Abdominal pain and mild fever may also be present.

It should be easy to understand why people with common migraine refer to their attacks as "sick headaches." Sometimes, when the intensity of the attack increases, fainting occurs, although it is not clear whether this is due simply to the headache pain or to other biological events that accompany it.

THE GENETICS OF MIGRAINE

Migraine is usually a genetic disorder, and so, it can be inherited. It is common for individuals with migraine to have other members of their family who have "sick headaches." Frequently, relatives have inappropriately presumed or have been told that their headaches are "sinus" or tension headaches. Occasionally members of one or two generations are spared, but a history of headaches in aunts, uncles, cousins, or grandparents is frequent.

THE MIGRAINE PERSONALITY

Certain personality features may be common among many of you who have migraine. This does not mean that *nerves* cause your headaches. What it does mean is that given the biological predisposition to have migraine, certain personality features may impose stress upon the individual and that it is the stress, not the personality features themselves, that may serve to trigger the painful attacks.

Many of you with migraine are perfectionistic, overly conscientious, and perhaps too rigid in your ways. You are meticulously neat and tidy, compulsive, and often very hard workers. It is likely that you are intelligent, exacting, and place a very high premium on success. You are probably very sensitive, too self-critical, and also much too concerned about what others think of you. You may have hostile or angry feelings toward relatives and others, but you cannot express these feelings openly. You are prone to overwork, fatigue, worry, and resentment. It is quite characteristic of you to react to stress and frustration with greater intensity than you should.

Of course many people who have elements of this personality profile do not have migraine, and many people with migraine do not have the features described. Migraine, like many other medical disorders, is not simply explained by any single, consistently present factor, or any of the various elements we have described. However, these personality features appear frequently and they perhaps in some way help trigger the development of the migraine syndrome in many of you.

At the end of this chapter you will find an informally designed exercise called the Migraine Personality Quiz. Those of you wishing to test your personality against the so-called migraine personality may find this exercise informative and entertaining.

WHEN MIGRAINE BEGINS

Migraine most frequently begins during the years between adolescence and the early twenties, although it is not uncommon for migraine to develop in childhood or after the age of forty. One of the interesting features of migraine is that some individuals may experience various nonheadache symptoms years before the actual headaches begin. For example, episodes of recurring vomiting in childhood, particularly at moments of excitement or anticipation, unexplained abdominal pain, and a tendency toward developing motion sickness are present in many people who go on to develop a more typical form of migraine later in their lives.

Migraine occurs more often in women than in men, and the peak years for migraine seem to be during the twenties and thirties. Some investigators believe that women are just more likely to seek medical care for their headaches than are men, thus biasing the statistics toward women. This does not seem likely to us. While the actual female-to-male ratio is difficult to determine, more women than men do suffer from migraine. No evidence of which we are aware suggests that this difference reflects a greater tendency for women to seek medical help.

FREQUENCY AND PATTERN OF MIGRAINE ATTACKS

Migraine is a transient disorder. This means that attacks are temporary, beginning and eventually ending without treatment. Occasionally headaches develop with such regularity that victims are able to predict precisely when the attacks will occur. This is commonly the case when migraine occurs during menstruation or on weekends, holidays, or during a particular time of sleep. Most often, however, migraine episodes occur without predictability and a recognizable pattern cannot be identified.

Attacks may develop as often as three or four times a week, once a month, or only once in several years. Some individuals experience a remission, with the attacks absent for ten to twenty years, only for the headaches to reappear again, decades later, in the same or a different pattern. The frequency of attacks may change with time, occasionally becoming more frequent during periods of increased stress and frustration.

Just as the frequency of attacks can change, the intensity of the attacks and their pattern can also change. For example, an adult who seeks medical attention for migraine often recalls that headaches of a less bothersome nature or of a completely different pattern were experienced in childhood, misbelieving that the migraine attacks are a recent problem, when in all probability, they are all part of the same headache condition.

EVENTS AND CIRCUMSTANCES THAT TRIGGER AN ATTACK

If you have migraine, you were probably born with a biological migraine predisposition. The frequency and nature of your attacks will be determined by what are called triggering factors. These triggering, or precipitating, factors range from emotionally charged situations to foods and drugs, certain kinds of visual effects, and weather or hormonal changes.

Aside from mere interest in such triggering phenomena, we believe that effective treatment and prevention require a thorough understanding of which headache-provoking circumstances are relevant to your case. Certain triggering factors are obvious; others remain obscure.

Emotions: Stress, Frustration, Depression, and Letdown—Emotions are a very important factor when considering the triggering of migraine attacks, even though emotional provocation is not always apparent to those who suffer from its influence. It is very common for migraines to worsen during periods of increasing pressure. The pressure to achieve what are often unreachable goals typically can lead to a series of attacks. Anger, particularly when not expressed, can trigger migraines. Intense mental concentration, such as studying for examinations, or a competitive business situation, may also be antecedent to headaches.

Some people who are prone to migraine experience attacks only *after* the emotionally distressing events have passed or lessened, rather than during the period of stress. This has been called letdown headache and can be one of the influential factors in provoking the weekend or holiday migraine. Some of our medical students claim that they invariably get headaches on the first or second days of their vacations rather than during the preparation for their examinations.

One psychiatric theory suggests that some illnesses like migraine actually represent the symbolic acting out of a psychological drama. The headache symbolically represents past or present (or even future) emotional events. For example, some psychiatrists believe that the wheezing in asthma allegedly represents a "crying out" or protest of separation from mother and womb. In the same way, the pounding headache of migraine is purported to be a symbolic enactment of "pounding" one's head, or perhaps that of someone else, against an immovable obstacle. We do not accept this speculative psychiatric theory; it does not seem to explain the majority of migraine attacks encountered in practice. Nevertheless, in some way not yet completely understood, emotional upset does indeed play a critical role in precipitating migraine in many patients.

While many physicians are quick to cite emotional disturbances as the cause of headache, many migraine victims do not have a history of significant emotional upset—except perhaps the stress of so often suffering from headache. In our experience, raising the issue of a possible emotional source for the headache early in the patient-doctor interaction, without thoroughly considering other possible triggering circumstances, can impair the creation of ideal patient-doctor communications. Many patients feel that their complaints are being dismissed when premature emphasis is placed on emotional factors.

Nevertheless, those who do not believe that emotional factors can cause changes in the body might consider the time that someone scratched/screeched fingernails on a blackboard, causing you to get goosebumps, or the time that someone used an embarrassing word and you blushed, or perhaps when some frightening event caused your heart to speed up, your brow to sweat, your stomach to cramp, and your hands to tremble. All of these represent significant *physiological* responses to *emotional* events. They represent not diseases but, for many people, normal and expected reactions. Current evidence suggests that chronic stress may indeed impose significant biochemical and physiological changes on the body. Patients with specific predispositions may indeed be more responsive to these emotionally induced physical changes than others.

Hormones, Hormonal Changes, and Pregnancy—Many women appear to experience migraine more intensely at times of hormonal change—menstruation, ovulation, menopause, or at the beginning or just following pregnancy. It is known that female hormones, either those occurring naturally (endogenous) or those ingested (exogenous), have emotional as well as biological influences upon the body, and about half of the women patients who have migraine believe that their attacks occur most frequently just before, during, or soon after their menstrual period.

Most women with migraine who take birth control pills or other female hormone preparations experience more frequent and more painful attacks of longer duration. When these agents are withdrawn, there is often a dramatic improvement in the patient's condition. Occasionally women will experience an ameliorating effect from these drugs.

It is our opinion that women with migraine, particularly the classical form, should not use birth control pills or other female hormone preparations unless there is an extraordinary medical reason to do so. Stroke and other serious illnesses occur more frequently when these substances are taken. Accumulating evidence suggests that the inconvenience encountered by not taking the pill may be worthwhile. When advised to discontinue birth control pills, some of our patients state that this action will succeed only in creating one "headache" in place of another!

The safety of taking hormones is a controversial medical issue. The hormones at the center of this debate are those in birth control pills, the agents used against menopausal symptoms, and diethylstilbestrol (DES), the agent used as the "morning-after pill." Reasonably sound evidence suggests that these hormones may place some women at greater than ordinary risk of developing certain diseases, such as stroke, heart attack, and cancer. Women who take these substances, and who also have migraine, may be placing themselves at even greater risk of developing stroke and heart attack than those who do not have migraine. Smoking may add an additional risk factor, so that a woman who has migraine, takes hormones, and smokes cigarettes may well be placing herself at considerably greater risk for developing these diseases than women who are not influenced by any of these factors.

There is an urgent need for additional scientific evidence regarding these issues. Learning a way to determine in advance which people are most apt to develop serious complications is particularly important, and until the evidence for or against the use of these hormones is conclusive, restraint is essential.

Pregnancy has a varying effect on migraine headache. There is a good chance that preexisting migraine will markedly improve after the first three months of pregnancy but return soon after delivery. However, some women with preexisting migraine experience a worsening throughout pregnancy, and still others say that at delivery, or the days immediately following delivery, their migraines first began.

Foods, Beverages, and Drugs—Some foods, beverages, and drugs can precipitate migraine in certain individuals. A quarter of our patients think that their headaches are influenced by what they eat or drink. The foods and beverages most often charged as offensive are fatty foods, cheese, alcohol, chocolate, citrus fruits (particularly oranges), monosodium glutamate (MSG), and nitrite-containing foods. Monosodium glutamate is found in many packaged foods, spices, seasonings, and canned foods. Nitrites are found in hot dogs and other smoked, preserved, or cured meats. The role of food and food additives and preservatives and their relationship to headache will be discussed more thoroughly in Chapter 9.

A migraine headache may also be precipitated by certain drugs, particularly those that lower blood pressure. Examples of this are reserpine and hydralazine, two agents found in many blood-pressure-lowering medications.

While some foods, beverages, and medications can provoke a migraine, missing meals can also trigger an attack. If your headaches occur during long periods without food or as a result of diets or fasts(five to six hours or more), you may be one of the people susceptible to an attack from this cause. Going without food from an early dinner hour the night before until breakfast the following day, about twelve to fourteen hours or more, may likewise provoke an attack. This does not necessarily mean that you have hypoglycemia, or low blood sugar.

An early-morning headache can sometimes be prevented by eating a low-carbohydrate snack just before bedtime. While eating a small snack between meals may be helpful in preventing attacks in some people, once the headache begins, eating may not have much effect. It is important to reemphasize that simply because headaches are triggered by missing meals or prevented by eating snacks prior to retiring, this does not imply, much less *prove,* that hypoglycemia is present. Most normal human beings can go weeks without food and, because of the body's ability to make sugar from its own protein and fat, maintain relatively normal blood sugar levels. During shorter fasts, say overnight, the body draws on its storage supply of sugar in the liver in order to maintain a normal blood level. It is believed that the *physiology* required to maintain normal blood sugar levels between meals, not hypoglycemia, may be the triggering factor. Perhaps by eating regularly, one eliminates the need for the appropriate physiological changes, thereby removing the trigger for the migraine attack.

Weather and Temperature Changes—Occasionally, changes of indoor or outdoor temperature, humidity, altitude, or atmospheric pressure can be the catalyst that provokes headaches. Some people notice that the sudden change in temperature when entering or leaving an air-conditioned room, or a sudden wind storm, will result in a headache.

The effects of atmospheric pressure and climate and their relationship to sickness have been of interest for centuries. "Ill winds" throughout the world have long been suspected of bringing on a variety of discomforts, including depression, irritability, respiratory ailments, and headaches. These winds are known in different parts of the world by various names, such as the Santa Ana of Southern California, the desert winds of Arizona, the *maltemia* of Greece, the *sharav* of Israel, the *foehn* of Switzerland, the the *bohorok* of Sumatra, and the *autun* of France.

A scientific study on the effects of the *sharav* in Israel* demonstrated a variety of biological changes in human beings during these weather fronts. Based on the evidence from this research, it was suggested that a change in the body's chemical balance can occur in some individuals who are exposed to this weather. This change was considered partially responsible for the physical discomfort, including headache, that can occur in association with changes in the weather.

When low-pressure weather fronts enter our area, many migraine patients who are free from headaches will again experience troublesome attacks. Falling temperatures and rising humidity are particularly likely to provoke migraine. The winter seems worse in this respect than the other seasons.

A number of patients have complained that the hot, dry air of a sauna provokes their headaches.

Weekend and Holiday Headaches—Some people are ashamed to admit that they experience headaches only on weekends, holidays, or when traveling. Sigmund Freud allegedly suffered from Sunday migraine. Bizarre as it may seem, weekend and holiday headaches are recognized entities. Nevertheless, they are likely to create cynical disbelief in family and friends. In some of you,

* F. G. Sulman, "Climatic Factors in the Incidence of Attacks of Migraine," in *Hemicrania* (1974), p. 2.

headaches usually do not occur during the week but can be reliably predicted whenever you are on a holiday or vacation.

Theories have been offered to explain this weekend and holiday migraine. One theory suggests that the weekend headache, migraine or otherwise, is related to caffeine withdrawal. Caffeine has a vasoconstricting effect, causing blood vessels to narrow. Ingesting too much caffeine can cause headaches, but withdrawal from excessive amounts can result in a widening of the blood vessels or vasodilation, which also causes headaches. For example, if you ordinarily consume large amounts of coffee or other caffeine-containing foods, beverages, and medications during weekdays and do not ingest a similar amount during the early mornings of weekends or holidays, a withdrawal rebound headache can result. Getting up at the same time on weekends as you do on weekdays and drinking coffee or other caffeine-containing beverages, as you usually do, may cut down on the severity of your headaches. But we recommend a different long-range treatment: discontinuance or at least control of the total caffeine intake rather than increasing it on weekends. This can most easily be done by gradually cutting down on the number of cups of coffee or tea you drink or the drugs you take.

A likely cause of many weekend or holiday headaches is altered sleep patterns, independent of caffeine. Migraines that begin during sleep may start during one of several stages of sleep. Of particular interest is the stage called Rapid Eye Movement sleep, or REM sleep. During this phase of sleep, a variety of biological events occurs, including dreaming, changes in muscle tone, and penile erection. In adults this stage of sleep accounts for approximately 25 percent of total sleeping time. It is of interest that when some people are experimentally deprived of REM sleep, a variety of psychiatric problems develops. With respect to headaches, however, prolonged sleeping and napping can result in headache because REM sleeping time is increased. In some of you, sleep is definitely a headache trigger. Arising on weekends at the same time as during the week can help avoid this reaction. Dr. James Dexter, a noted headache authority, has done much of the exciting research that has enhanced our understanding of sleep patterns and their relationship to headaches.

Additional theories for weekend headaches consider biological as well as emotional factors. Late-night hours, alcohol, parties, smoke-filled rooms, and increased social or sexual demands cannot be overlooked. The weekend or holiday headache may also reflect a "letdown" phenomenon, which, as we have already discussed, may also cause a headache.

Exertion—Some people experience attacks only during or after physical exertion. Jogging, jumping rope, and playing tennis are often cited. It is possible that the headaches related to exertion may be caused by either the chemical or blood vessel changes that occur during physical exertion or perhaps by the depletion of certain biological substances following the exercise. Perhaps related are the severe headaches that occur in some people, particularly men, at the time of sexual orgasm. This troubling condition is called benign orgasmic cephalagia and will be discussed in Chapter 7.

Other Triggering Events—A variety of other factors can trigger migraine. Among these are light-related influences, like glaring artificial light or sunlight, flickering light from a television set, or moving pictures. Some people are sensitive to motion, especially the often jarring quality of automobile or train travel. In some people the combination of flickering lights and motion is particularly irritating. Many of our patients have told us that sunlight flickering through trees or off water is a particularly provoking stimulus. Airplane travel can also cause throbbing headaches in many individuals. This may be related to changes in cabin pressure.

"Hypertension" is a term that means high blood pressure. There is some evidence that people with migraine may be more likely to develop hypertension than nonmigraine people. If hypertension becomes severe, migraine attacks can be triggered. And many of the medications used to treat hypertension, particularly drugs containing reserpine, hydralazine, and some of the diuretics, can provoke headaches—migraine or other varieties.

During the winter, faulty furnaces that emit into the house products of combustion can cause headaches in some ways similar to migraine. This should be at least suspected in individuals free from headaches except in cold months.

Individuals who either visit or live in highly elevated locations, such as mountain areas, can experience migraine-like headaches as a consequence of the rarefied atmosphere and the reduction of oxygen, which causes a biological compensation in your blood and blood vessels.

In a similar way, smoking may provoke migraine-like headaches in patients with the vascular headache predisposition. Research has indicated many biological changes in the blood and blood vessels of smokers. Many patients will report an improvement in their headaches when smoking cigarettes is curtailed. Some patients state that just being in a smoke-filled room will trigger an attack.

Before leaving the subject of elements that trigger migraine, we suggest that if your migraines unexpectedly worsen, you might consider the following as possible explanations:

Recent use of birth control pills or other hormones.
Elevation of blood pressure.
An emotional state of anxiety, depression, or stress.
Overuse of the medications that are prescribed for headache treatment, including caffeine, pain killers, or ergot compounds.
A recent change in eating habits, including missing meals.

Unfortunately, the true explanation of why your headaches have worsened usually remains a mystery.

THE COURSE, OR NATURAL HISTORY, OF MIGRAINE

The natural history of a disease is the expected course the disease will take when a medical cure is unavailable. Since migraine is treatable but not curable, its natural history is important. The course of migraine may follow many patterns, but most of you who have migraine will experience attacks at varying intervals throughout most of your lifetime. Although there are many exceptions, middle age often brings a welcome decrease in both the severity and frequency of migraine headaches.

While many women experience a dramatic improvement in their attacks as they enter and complete their menopausal years, some unfortunate people suffer a dramatic worsening of attacks during or after the menopause. In some of these women, hormones given for the symptoms of menopause seem to trigger the headaches. In a few cases, the hormones seem to help.

MIGRAINE IN CHILDREN

Children may have migraine, and approximately one-fourth of our adult patients suffered from migraine during childhood. A major problem in assessing the incidence of migraine in children is that the symptoms are often different from those in the adult, with headache often being an inconspicuous part of the syndrome.

Although migraine headaches as severe as those in adults may be present in a child, very different symptoms may exist. The most striking features of childhood migraine are often episodes of abdominal pain, unexplained nausea and vomiting, listlessness, fever, and painful sensitivity to sunlight. Frequently these attacks precede or follow an exciting or tense event. In some children, stomach complaints are so severe and frequent that serious illnesses, such as appendicitis, are considered.

Childhood migraine may continue into adult forms or may terminate sometime in adolescence. It is interesting to note that the childhood form of migraine strikes both males and females equally, whereas in the adult population migraine occurs much more frequently in the female population. There are many possible explanations for this, but the exact reason why this change in incidence occurs is not fully understood.

The personality of children with migraine is often similar to that of an adult with migraine. These children are frequently intelligent, shy, and perfectionist. Not uncommonly, their parents are educated and successful and often impose, quite unintentionally, unreasonable pressures for achievement on their offspring, who would ordinarily perform well in school anyway. These children are easily frustrated, tense, and high strung. In some families, children tend to be discouraged from any showing of anger, even when it may be appropriate.

Children with migraine may have slight abnormalities detectable by electroencephalography. The abnormal changes are in some respects similar to those found in epilepsy. The significance of this remains controversial, but it is of considerable interest that some children with migraine will improve when placed on anti-seizure medications like phenytoin (Dilantin).

It is very important to recognize that when children are in pain, parents may show more love, responsibilities may be lessened, and expectations for performance may be reduced. These create a certain advantage to having pain, a phenomenon generally termed *secondary gain.* It is our opinion that it is vitally important that physicians or other health professionals treating young people in pain counsel not only the patient, but also the family.

If a child begins to appreciate too frequently the "power" of illness, it may well influence his/her personality, character, and relationships with other people. Once this happens and pain becomes a component of the way an individual relates to his/her world, influencing relationships, educational efforts, and other important decisions, then successful treatment of this problem will require much more than simple treatment for headaches.

THE TREATMENT OF MIGRAINE

Chronic headaches, such as migraine, in which there is no injured tissue to account for the symptoms, can be *treated* but not *cured.* Pain of a migraine and muscle contraction headache, as well as the other chronic headache disorders, is most likely a reaction of normal tissue to various physiological or psychological events. It cannot be treated as can a wart, an infection, or a tumor. There is no surgery, antibiotic, or other specific therapy that can "heal" or remove the injured tissue. The tissue is not primarily abnormal. What must be attempted is to control the symptoms, and this can be effectively achieved in most individuals.

Treating Your Own Migraine Without Medications—Most severe migraine attacks require medication for relief, but there are some simple nondrug therapies that may help to prevent the headache or retard the frequency and severity of your attacks. The following suggestions may be helpful in preventing migraine attacks, but do not assume you have migraine unless a physician has established the diagnosis.

1. Discontinue or avoid any circumstances, events, foods, over-the-counter medications, or beverages that you feel could have precipitated your attacks.

2. If your headaches seem to be related to the use of birth control pills or other prescription medications, discuss the matter with a physician before discontinuing them.

3. Learn to relax and to reduce stress; make sure that each day you have at least one-half hour to yourself for thorough relaxation.

4. Engage regularly in enjoyable hobbies and relaxing activities.

5. Unless exercise is known to provoke your attacks, regular physical exercise is advisable, providing your health is good.

6. Avoid sleeping late. In fact, get up as early as possible each day and avoid daytime napping.

7. Biofeedback and behavior modifications appear to be worthwhile in some cases of migraine. In fact, after adequate screening by a physician, biofeedback may be the treatment of choice for children and young people with migraine. Biofeedback and behavior modification can be learned from qualified professionals and we encourge this treatment in many patients because it imposes no health risk, and therefore deserves special respect. Other similar efforts, such as yoga and transcendental meditation, may also be useful.

8. Learn to express your feelings. Try to speak your mind and express yourself outwardly and frankly. We have already suggested that migraine may occur when hostility, anger, and guilt are pent up and simmering inside. Open the door to these feelings and let them escape. You will feel better.

9. If you are troubled by migraines on weekends, holidays, or during vacations, reappraise your indulgences, like sleeping late,

too much coffee, cocktail parties, and spicy or preserved foods, and go to bed and get up on weekends the same time you normally do on weekdays.

10. Many patients state that they have fewer headaches after they have quit smoking. It is possible that the products of combustion play a role in dilating arteries. This may result from the body's attempt to get more blood to the brain when challenged by the oxygen reduction or other elements in the polluted air.

Treating Your Own Attacks Once They Have Begun—We do not know of any treatment, medication or otherwise, that consistently and effectively relieves the migraine attack once it has begun. Many of our patients tell us that an attack will end only after it has run its course. If you develop a migraine headache, you may want to try one of a number of nonmedical remedies. We have accumulated a short list of home-style treatments that have been suggested to us by our patients and friends. Some are reasonable and may have a scientific basis. A few defy any logic, but those who have given us these ideas claim that they work. Here they are. Use your own judgment in their application, and certainly avoid anything that seems unpleasant.

1. Apply cold compresses (moist or dry) to the head and neck. Most migraine sufferers, prefer cold to heat, but you might try heat to the back of the neck and cold to the top of the head. The heat usually relieves the muscle contraction in the neck region that can be a response to the pain in your head.

2. Apply pressure to your temples with your palms or a firm object such as a cold washcloth that has been tightly folded. (The technique of acupressure can be learned from available literature.)

3. Retreat to a quiet, darkened room; place your head higher than the rest of your body; try to relax and sleep.

4. If you are nauseated, try to vomit. This reduces the headache in a few patients. (Avoid this if you have any disorder of your digestive system.)

5. Try crying vigorously. Several patients claim that this helps considerably, but others claim that it intensifies their pain.

6. Fill a basin with ice cubes and cold water and thrust your arms or the top of your head into the basin (see below).

7. Immerse your entire body in cold water. Then before drying, stand in front of a fan or an air conditioner for a short time. A friend who uses a variation of this told us she throws on her clothes and runs outside into the cold with her hair dripping wet.

These are only examples of therapeutic anecdotes, efforts devised by individuals to treat their own headaches, and do not imply any endorsement by us. Indeed, some, such as the cold water techniques, may be downright dangerous especially in patients with high blood pressure or heart disease.

Treating Migraine with Medications—Ideally, it would be safer to treat symptoms without having to resort to taking medications, all of which possess some potential risk. Currently, however, most migraine patients require medicine in order to achieve the maximum possible relief.

We are eager to teach you about these drugs, including their potential side effects. There is no such thing as an entirely safe medication, but then there is very little in today's world that is entirely safe, and this includes the water we drink, the air we breathe, and the cars we drive. What must clearly be emphasized, however, is that carefully administered medications, monitored by qualified physicians, impose relatively few unacceptable risks when used for the appropriate reasons. Like all things in life, important "trade-offs" must be made, and treating pain is no exception.

We believe that it is important for physicians to carefully inform their patients about commonly encountered side effects. This, however, creates a "double-edged sword." On the one hand, advising patients of potential hazards of their medication enhances their own ability to monitor their health. On the other hand, suggesting to certain patients that such unwanted effects are possible may add to the patient's anxiety and may even "predispose" the patient to unwanted effects. We believe that, on balance, most patients benefit from such knowledge.

The general categories of drugs used to treat headache include analgesics, mood-altering drugs, and specific agents for migraine and other headaches. Some drugs are designed to be taken to stop (abort) the occasional headache, while others are used daily to prevent the frequent headache from beginning. The advantage of the abortive approach is that it requires the use of medications only when the attack occurs. The disadvantage of this approach, however, is that the drugs cannot be taken frequently. Furthermore, the preheadache phase of classical migraine escapes control with the abortive approach. The preventive approach, on the other hand, is best for frequently occurring attacks. The advantage of this therapy is that when successfully employed, the migraine is prevented from developing. The disadvantage is that medication must be taken daily, much like birth control pills to prevent conception.

ABORTIVE TREATMENT: For mild, infrequent migraine, simple analgesics, like aspirin and acetaminophen, may occasionally effectively and safely abort the pain, but analgesics should not be taken daily for headaches. Sometimes, a sedative or a sleeping pill can help the victim sleep through the several hours of discomfort.

Unfortunately, analgesics, even the narcotic type given by injection, are not always effective in relieving migraine, and many people cannot afford the luxury of sleeping. Recently we suggested sleeping for a housewife who has occasional migraine. She quickly responded, "How can you expect me to take the afternoon off when I have three screaming kids? They'll destroy my house!"

Although these drugs are of value in some circumstances, most patients with migraine need special medications that exert some control of blood vessels. Various forms of the so-called vasoactive medications (medications that affect blood vessels) can be used in either the abortive approach (to stop an attack) or the preventive approach (to prevent the onset of an attack).

Ergotamine is the most commonly employed specific agent to abort a migraine. Ergotamine is often combined with caffeine, sedatives, and antinauseants. Ergotamine can be administered in ordinary tablet form, inserted in the rectum as a suppository, used as a tablet that dissolves under the tongue, given as an inhalant to be breathed into the lungs, or injected. To be most effective, the ergotamine preparations must be taken at the very first sign of migraine. In the case of classical migraine, this means during the preheadache phase. This requires that the drug be constantly available. The unpleasant preheadache phase of classical migraine, which announces that a headache will follow, is, naturally, not prevented by ergotamine since the drug's major effect is to combat the painful dilation of the blood vessels and not the constriction associated with the preheadache phase. This is a serious shortcoming of the abortive medications because it is the preheadache phase and its potential permanent neurological symptoms that pose the greatest medical risk.

There is some evidence to suggest that vasoconstricting medications, when given during the preheadache phase, may actually impose an additional risk toward stroke. We advise our patients with classic migraine either not to take vasoconstrictive drugs at all or to delay their use until the preheadache phase has terminated. While this reduces the potential effectiveness of the drug by delaying its entrance into the bloodstream, we believe that the reduction in therapeutic effectiveness is worth the enhanced safety that this delay affords.

The major failings of this widely used and frequently successful abortive approach include the need to have the medication available at all times, the inability to prevent the preheadache symptoms, and the potential unwanted reactions associated with ergotamine's use.

Usually a medication capable of producing beneficial effects can also be responsible for side reactions, some equally as troublesome as the primary complaint. Were you to read the list of adverse and potentially dangerous side effects of simple aspirin, you might shudder to think that such a drug could be used without a prescription or medical supervision. A basic principle governing the use of any medication is that the possible benefits must be carefully weighed against the possible risks.

Fortunately, most of the side reactions associated with the medications used for migraine are relatively mild and usually disappear when the drug is withdrawn. Nevertheless, ergotamine should not be taken by people with blood vessel disorders, such as coronary artery disease and high blood pressure, or with significantly impaired liver or kidney function, or during pregnancy. The reason for abstaining during pregnancy is that ergotamine may directly affect the uterus and its blood vessels.

The most common adverse reactions associated with ergotamine are nausea and vomiting, often symptoms of the migraine itself. Other adverse effects include leg cramps, numbness and tingling of the fingers and toes, chest pain, abnormal heart rate, and itching and swelling of extremities. These drugs can be given safely only once or twice a week, and they are not recommended when migraine occurs more frequently. When these drugs are taken regularly, dangerous narrowing of blood vessels may occur. Rebound widening of blood vessels often develops when the medication's effect wears off. Taking more medication will improve the rebound headache, but a dangerous cycle of dependency can lead to serious consequences.

The unwanted effects of ergotamine, including severe constriction of arteries, may be intensified with fever or significant infection. Patients taking ergotamine should either reduce their dosage or avoid the use of this drug during such episodes.

The following are some of the preparations containing ergot derivatives used in the abortive approach to treatment: Cafergot (tablet or suppository form), Ergomar and Ergostat (under the tongue—sublingual form), Ergotamine Medihaler (inhalant), Migral (tablet form), and Wigraine (tablet or suppository form).

In Canada, ergotamine is found in many of the same preparations as in the United States. In addition, a Canadian preparation available in capsule form, called Gravergol, contains ergotamine, an antinauseant (dimenhydrinate) and caffeine. Dimenhydrinate (Gravol in Canada, Dramamine in the United States) is also available alone as an antinauseant.

Midrin is a combination tablet (vasoactive, analgesic, and sedative substance) also used for abortive relief of migraine. The active antimigraine agent in this product is isometheptene mucate and is not marketed by itself, but only in combination. Although isometheptene may cause some of the same side reactions as ergotamine and has many of the same precautionary restrictions, it is our experience that it is usually well tolerated by most people for mild-to-moderate migraine. Its effectiveness is sometimes enhanced by the simultaneous administration of two aspirin.

It is also possible to abort a migraine with the use of drugs called phenothiazines. This group of medicines known as major tranquilizers have been used primarily for psychoses and for control of nausea. They may exert control over pain in a way quite independent of its other effects. We have found that chlorpromazine (Thorazine), which has both tranquilizing and antinauseant effects, can be very helpful in some patients.

The abortive drugs are used to treat an individual attack. Combinations of analgesics, sedatives, antinauseants, and specific antimigraine drugs are sometimes necessary.

PREVENTIVE TREATMENT WITH MEDICATIONS: When the frequency of the attacks precludes the safe use of the abortive antimigraine drugs, analgesics, and sedatives, the preventive approach becomes justifiable. These preventive medications can be taken daily without the same risks associated with daily use of abortive medications, although these drugs, as with all medications, possess potential hazards.

Mood-altering drugs—antidepressants and tranquilizers—are sometimes beneficial either alone or in combination with other medications when the headache frequency justifies a preventive approach. As mentioned above, it may not be the mechanism by which the medication tranquilizes or reduces depression that is important in controlling pain. Current evidence suggests that these drugs exert an influence on pain perception, independent of their other effects.

Current research has suggested that certain of the antidepressants, particularly amitriptyline (Elavil, Endep), may exert an antimigraine effect when taken daily, independent of any direct effect on mood.

Amitriptyline (Endep and Elavil), an antidepressant, has many effects upon the body, and its use requires occasional blood tests and physical examinations. Common side effects include dryness of the mouth, blurriness of vision, dizziness, sedation, tingling in the extremities, and various other symptoms (including weight gain) that your doctor should discuss with you. The drug should not be taken by persons with some forms of glaucoma, urination problems, or those who are taking certain other medications. Pregnant women should not take this drug.

Amitriptyline taken in relatively small dosages at bedtime may have an impressive effect in the prevention of muscle contraction pain as well. Amitriptyline can be used in conjunction with other migraine drugs.

Most individuals taking this drug experience few, if any, serious side reactions, and it is fast becoming an accepted adjunct in headache prevention.

Cyproheptadine (Periactin) possesses antihistamine properties, and it also counteracts the chemical serotonin, the substance that plays an important role in migraine. Cyproheptadine should not be taken if you have glaucoma or asthma, or by any patient who is pregnant or has urinary or certain stomach conditions. It should never be taken at the same time you are using certain antidepressant drugs, and you should avoid this drug if you are elderly or debilitated. Antihistamines may induce seizures in some children with epilepsy and, therefore, must be used cautiously if there is a history of epilepsy. This drug may be particularly apt to produce adverse reactions when combined with alcohol or any depressant medication. Common undesirable effects of cyproheptadine include drowsiness and a feeling of dizziness and unsteadiness. Many patients complain of increased appetite and subsequent weight gain. Nevertheless, cyproheptadine is considered by many headache authorities to be a safe and effective drug for many headache types, particularly childhood migraine.

Bellergal, a compound drug, includes small amounts of ergotamine, a barbiturate tranquilizer, and an antinauseant. Because Bellergal contains such a small amount of ergotamine, it may be given daily for several months without significant risk of producing toxicity. But, as with other medications containing ergotamine, you should not use it if you have blood vessel or coronary artery disease, high blood pressure, kidney or liver disorders, or if you are pregnant. Because many antinauseants have an adverse effect on glaucoma, this drug should not be used by anyone suspected of having or known to have this condition. The most common side effects of Bellergal include dry mouth, drowsiness, and blurred vision.

Propranolol (Inderal), a medication that blocks the effect of the body's adrenalin on certain tissues, has now become recognized as an important drug in the prevention of migraine. Numerous studies, as well as current clinical experience, have shown impressive benefit in many patients. Propranolol is also being used for certain heart conditions, high blood pressure, and some other medical disorders as well. Propranolol cannot be used if you have asthma, severe allergic conditions, significantly slowed heart rate, very low blood pressure, uncontrolled diabetes, severe hypoglycemia, heart failure, or if you are pregnant.

During treatment with propranolol, your heart, blood pressure, and pulse rate should be watched and evaluated regularly. Although this drug is generally very well tolerated, some of the potential side effects include fatigue and gastrointestinal disturbances. Mild weight gain and some fluid accumulation have been reported. Unlike many other medications that are helpful against migraine, propranolol does not usually sedate the patients using it.

Methysergide (Sansert) simulates the action of serotonin, the chemical we have previously mentioned as important in the production of migraine headaches. This drug can be potentially hazardous when taken regularly for a prolonged time. It can produce scar formations in various organs, including the heart, lung, and around the kidneys. Methysergide can impair blood circulation to the extremities, and it can cause blood abnormalities and muscle cramps. Chest and abdominal pains, stomach upset, insomnia, dizziness, and hallucinations may also occur. These reactions understandably limit the usefulness of methysergide. However, most complications are reversible when the drug is withdrawn or the dose is reduced. You should not take this drug during pregnancy, or if you have poor circulation, heart disease, high blood pressure, or lung, liver, or kidney trouble. Despite its risks, methysergide has proved to be a very effective preventive antimigraine drug in many individuals. Most of the serious hazards of the drug can be avoided if it is used for only three or four months at a time and is then followed by a one- or two-month "drug holiday" in which no methysergide is taken.

It may come as a surprise to you that aspirin is mentioned in a list of preventive medications, since it is a simple analgesic and frequently fails to abort the already present migraine. But as we said earlier, current research in migraine is focusing on the possible higher-than-average risk of heart attacks and strokes in some migraine patients, particularly those with the classical migraine type. This risk may have something to do with increased platelet stickiness (platelets are clotting particles in the blood). Among aspirin's medical properties is an antiplatelet, anticlotting action. In experimental settings, aspirin is being given daily (one to two tablets per day) along with other drugs to combat this increased platelet stickiness. It remains to be seen whether aspirin has a reliable and beneficial effect on this problem or on preventing, as opposed to aborting, the headache of migraine.

Clonidine (Catapres) is yet another drug used to prevent migraine. It is used primarily as an agent to control high blood pressure, but effectiveness in controlling migraine has been suggested by some medical reports. Side effects include dry mouth and drowsiness. Mild gastrointestinal distress, weight gain, and vivid dreaming are also reported. The drug should be reduced slowly when discontinued. Use during pregnancy should be avoided.

The substance pizotifen (Sandomigran) is not available in the United States but is in Canada. This substance has serotonin-blocking properties and other effects on the amines. Although we do not have personal experience with the drug, scientific reports suggest effective control of migraine in many patients. The most common side effects reported have been weight gain and fatigue. The drug is related to cyproheptadine and some of the antidepressants, and as with these and all drugs, its use during pregnancy must be avoided.

We have discussed the important precautions concerning the use of some of these medications, along with a few of their potential side effects, because we wish to emphasize to you once again that most medications are potentially hazardous, whether they require a prescription or not. Nevertheless, when taken with caution and with regular medical supervision, these medications can make the life of a migraine patient more enjoyable. The adverse reactions we have mentioned, particularly the serious ones, may have occurred in only a small percentage of the many thousands of people who have safely taken these drugs. Most of these medications will not produce significant adverse reactions in the vast majority of people. Nevertheless, it is best to avoid medication whenever possible. When their use is necessary, you should be alert to the possible consequences, even though serious adverse reactions are relatively unlikely.

Finally, the most important element in the successful treatment of migraine is the development of a trusting professional relationship between you and your physician. Your doctor must be devoted to the relief of your distress and not become frustrated or offended by the failure of any initial therapy. It may take months of trying one treatment after another until you and your doctor discover one that will work for you. Your doctor must be willing to maintain close professional contact with you during this time. For your part, you must find a physician whom you trust and be willing to allow the time necessary to devise a "tailor-made" therapy that takes into account the pattern of your headaches, your personality, and your general health. Your interaction with the physician must be frank, open, and detailed, so that the medical as well as the emotional features of your problem are fully understood and confronted. While you should never invest blind faith in a physician, the development of a mutually trusting relationship creates the atmosphere essential for successful therapy.

Most of you can be helped considerably. In some migraine patients, the headaches have become so much a part of their lives that no matter how disruptive and distressing they are, removing the headaches is like removing a part of the body or altering the personality. Understandably, simply administering a drug is not alone the answer.

A SUMMARY OF THE BASIC FEATURES OF MIGRAINE

Episodes of headaches lasting hours to days and sometimes hurting on one side more than another.
Often begins in childhood, teens, or early twenties.
The presence of additional symptoms, including nausea and

vomiting, visual abnormalities, and sometimes weakness and numbness.

Often is inherited and other family members have similar headaches.

Attacks triggered by emotional factors, alcohol, certain foods, menstrual periods, exertion, weather changes, and sleep (attacks can awaken patients during the night).

During an attack, patients seek quiet, dark solitude.

After an attack, patients may feel "washed out" for hours or days.

A MIGRAINE PERSONALITY QUIZ

The so-called migraine personality is characterized by compulsive, perfectionistic, and self-critical tendencies. Often these features reflect an upbringing that placed a high premium on discipline, restraint, achievement, and respect for authority.

It is a matter of debate whether having the migraine personality really means that you are more likely to have migraine headaches. Certainly many migraine sufferers do not have these personality traits, and many people who have the migraine personality do not suffer from headaches.

The following exercise may help you determine whether or not some of the features of the migraine personality are present within you. The quiz is informal and is offered for your entertainment. To take this quiz, read each statement carefully and decide to what extent it applies to you. If the statement reflects your personality, write the number (3) as the score. Give the statement a score of (2) if it is rather like you but not exactly. Assign a score of (1) if the statement only minimally reflects your behavior. If the statement is not at all like you, give it a score of (0).

Score

1. You put a very high premium on neatness. You feel uncomfortable when things around you are out of place. You often find yourself rearranging things so they look neat and tidy.   ____

2. Even though you don't like to admit it, you are often angry at various people and situations. _____

3. Frequently your patience is quite thin. You make every effort to maintain self-control and seem calm on the surface, but you are really steaming inside. _____

4. Disapproval is very troubling to you. You make every effort to stand out and excel in the things you do. To you, being average at anything is almost the same as failure. _____

5. You become annoyed very easily at people who are not like you. Although you would like to change their ways, you become particularly incensed if they try to control you or change your manner. _____

6. Small irritations, such as ashes dropped on your table or people around who are messy, make you feel annoyed, hurt, or actually angry.

7. You are a *pleaser*. You often go out of your way to please and befriend individuals whom you either do not particularly like or who do not deserve the benefits of your efforts. Nevertheless, you choose to satisfy other people's needs at the neglect of your own. _____

8. You believe that working hard is a virtue, and you have little respect for people who do not share the philosophy that hard work is the price of achievement. _____

9. You constantly write lists. You makes lists for shopping, trips, birthdays, daily activities, and bills. You even write lists to remember what to tell your doctor or a friend. _____

10. Quite often you imagine yourself "telling people off." Nevertheless, you never seem to say these things to the right people at the right time. _____

11. You have a great deal of difficulty expressing your anger or disappointment. You end up smiling approvingly rather than exposing your true emotions or actually confronting anyone. _____

12. You tend to believe that your way is the best way. When a different approach is suggested, you are usually un-

willing to change, despite the possible merits or advantages. ____

13. You seldom take shortcuts, even if it means reaching your goal more simply or quickly. ____

14. You are extraordinarily organized. When given a responsibility, you create a plan to achieve your task efficiently. You will not rest comfortably until your goal is accomplished. ____

15. You place a very high premium on being on time. You are punctual about everything. You avoid being late even by a few minutes. You become very uncomfortable if you are tardy, even if there is an understandable reason. ____

16. You are concerned about bodily cleanliness and neatness. You are concerned about cleanliness and neatness in general. ____

17. You worry that you have a body odor or germs and find yourself washing, brushing your teeth, showering, or bathing probably more often than truly necessary. ____

18. You perform many little rituals that are part of your daily routine. For example, before going to bed at night you might perform certain tasks, often in a certain sequence, like making sure the front door is locked (even if you know it is), making sure objects are in their appropriate place, seeing that every knob on the stove is checked at least once (maybe even twice), or closing the closet door tightly. If you are prevented from carrying out these little rituals, you become upset and may not be able to fall asleep. ____

19. You disapprove of any form of procrastination. You must do things now! You live by the adage "Don't put off until tomorrow what you can do today." ____

20. When going out for an evening, you *must* be dressed appropriately and in the expected manner. Not being so makes you uncomfortable and very self-conscious. ____

21. Dirt is definitely your enemy. If you set out to clean

Score

something, you work to get every last particle of dirt removed.

     ——

22. When you have friends over to visit, everything must be in its proper place and very clean. For example, if an ashtray has a few ashes in it, you feel inclined to empty it repeatedly, even during the visit. You worry about what people might think of you if everything is not just so.

     ——

23. Your parents were very strict with you, insisting upon discipline, early toilet training, and a heavy emphasis on neatness, withholding of emotions, and on achievement.

24. Your handwriting is very neat. For you to be comfortable, things around you must also be very neat and orderly.

     ——

25. You are very critical of yourself. If you achieve something that you know was done well, you might nevertheless be inclined to deny its merits when complimented. Although you criticize yourself readily, you shun criticism from others and become angry and hurt if people question your actions.

     ——

26. You are a perfectionist. You enjoy being told that you are a perfectionist and consider it a fine compliment.

     ——

27. You are often constipated. Not only do you hold your emotions inside, but you hold on to everything. You do not let go of anything very easily.

     ——

28. You are a collector and a saver. Throwing something out is most difficult for you. You acquire much more than you actually need.

     ——

Add up your responses to determine your total score.

63–84: If your total score is in this range, you clearly possess features of the migraine personality. It is likely that your compulsive personality brings you a good deal of discomfort. You would probably benefit from any effort that would loosen up your compulsive, rigid life-style, but do not go about changing your life-style in a compulsive manner!

42–62: Your performance indicates that significant elements of the migraine personality are present in you. Whether or not you have migraine, you might consider loosening some of your more compulsive habits. You might feel better as a result.

21–41: Your score indicates that you have a reasonable balance between compulsive and noncompulsive elements in your personality.

0–20: Based on this quiz, you do not have much evidence of compulsiveness in your personality. If your life-style is disorganized and unstructured and if you find yourself suffering the consequences of unfulfilled ambitions, irresponsibility, and inability to achieve, you might consider becoming a bit more compulsive and organized in your ways. However, if you are happy—wonderful!

It occurs to us that if you are married or living with someone whose score on this test differs from yours by 40 or more points, you have ample reason for headaches—migraine or otherwise!

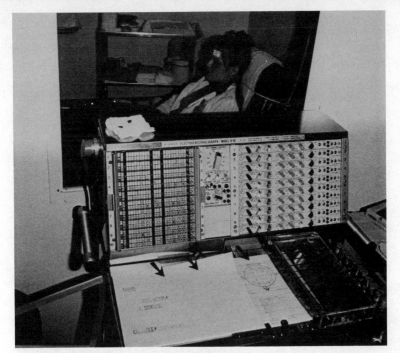

Photograph 1—**An Electroencephalograph.**

In the foreground is the electroencephalograph machine. The arrows point to the paper upon which the electroencephalogram is recorded. Behind the screen is seated the person undergoing the test. Electrodes are pasted to various locations on her scalp.

Photograph 2—**An Electroencephalogram.**

This is one segment taken from an electroencephalogram of an individual with a seizure disorder. On the left side of the tracing are seen large waves indicating seizure activity (see arrows). In the middle of this page of the tracing, more normal brain waves suddenly appear. Each line of the recording represents a different area of the brain; a survey of many regions can be studied by the electroencephalogram.

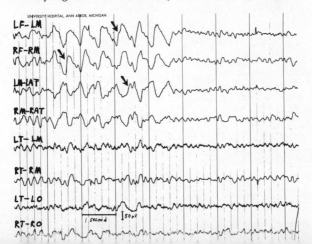

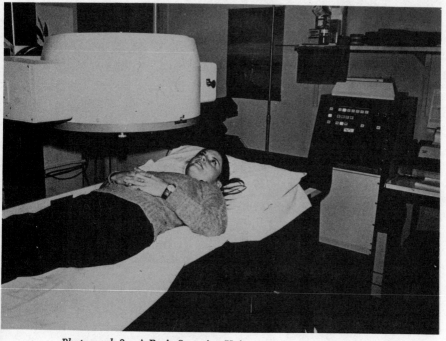

Photograph 3—A Brain-Scanning Unit.
    This photograph demonstrates the manner in which a brain scan is performed. Following the injection of the contrast material, the individual is placed under the scanning unit, which records the radioactivity in various locations of the brain.

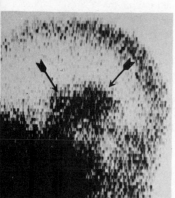

Photograph 4—A Brain Scan.
    The dark area (see arrows) represents abnormal "uptake," which in this particular case turned out to be a large brain tumor. (This patient *did not* have a headache.)

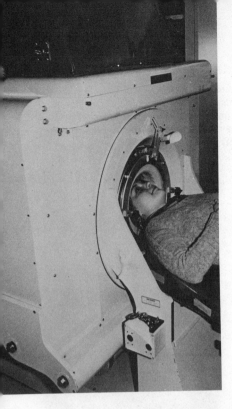

Photograph 5—**A Computerized Axial Tomography (CAT) Scanning Unit.**
This photograph shows a large "CAT" scanning unit. The machine rotates in a clockwise direction around the head of the individual undergoing the test.

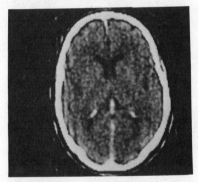

Photograph 6—**A CAT Scan.**
The "slice" of brain (gray substance) pictured here shows only one of many such views taken during the scanning procedure. The white rim around the brain is the skull. You are looking down from above, and the top of the picture represents the front. The dark structures looking like boomerangs are portions of the ventricles, which are only partially visible in this "slice" of the brain.

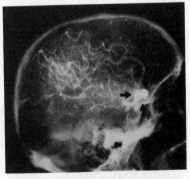

Photograph 7—**An Angiogram.**
The angiogram demonstrates the many blood vessels within and on the surface of the brain. Each vessel is filled with contrast material that, moments before, had been injected into the bloodstream. There are numerous abnormalities in this picture. The arrows point to blood vessel dilations—called aneurysms—which, in this individual, bled into and around the brain.

Photographs A–F

The following photographs represent a variety of visual abnormalities that can accompany migraine headaches, particularly the classical migraine. In most cases, these abnormalities are temporary. The photographs demonstrate what you would see were you to have one of these abnormalities.

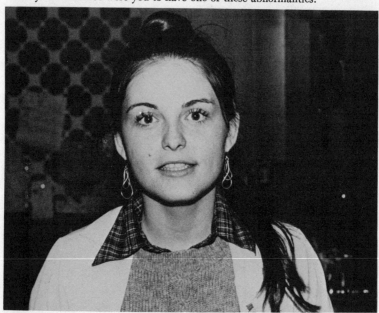

Photograph A—A picture of a woman as seen normally.

Photograph B—A large, glaring blind spot, negative scotoma, is present; this is what you would see, looking at the woman, if you had a negative scotoma. In migraine, a negative scotoma may locate anywhere in the visual field and may "travel" across the visual panorama during the preheadache phase.

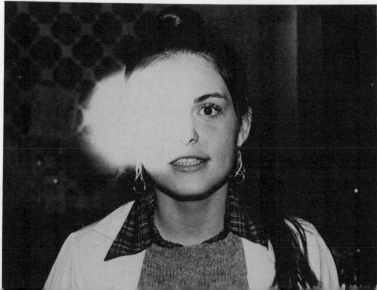

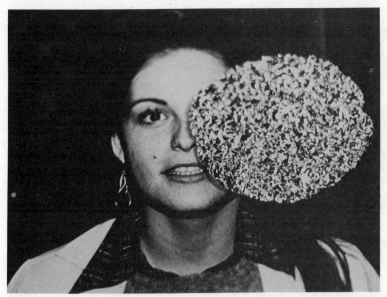

Photograph C—This is an attempt to photographically reproduce what is called a scintillating scotoma. Instead of an absence of vision, in a scintillating scotoma there is a glittering pattern in what would have been an area of blindness. In both cases, the area of the scotoma is effectively blinded. The picture is also slightly out of focus, demonstrating the blurred vision that commonly accompanies migraine headaches.

Photograph D—This photograph depicts loss of vision on an entire side of the visual field. When an entire half of the visual field is involved, the abnormality is called a hemianopsia (hemi-, half, -anopsia, without vision). This particular loss of vision is the fortification spectrum abnormality, a form experienced by many migraine patients; there are many varieties of this zigzag blindness. The area may be small or may involve the entire half of the visual field. In the left lower corner of this picture is a negative scotoma.

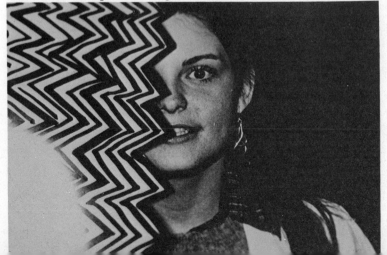

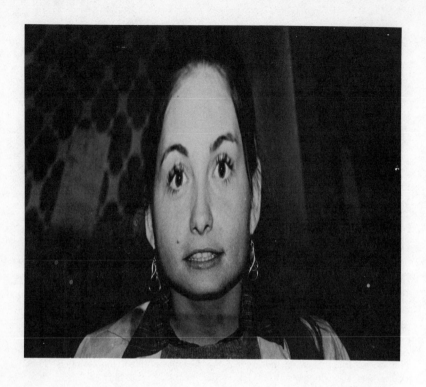

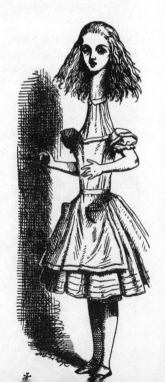

Photographs E and F—These two photographs demonstrate the distorted visual images that occur in the "Alice in Wonderland syndrome." Photograph E shows an elongated facial appearance on our lady model. Photograph F is taken directly from the book *Alice's Adventures in Wonderland*. The original drawings from Lewis Carroll's classic works were done by John Tenniel with Lewis Carroll's assistance.

Chapter **3** Muscle Contraction (Tension) Headaches

THE MUSCLE CONTRACTION (TENSION) HEADACHE PROFILE

The Muscle Contraction (Tension) Headache Profile below is a description of the symptoms of muscle contraction (tension) headaches. It is followed by a series of questions that a physician might ask you if muscle contraction headaches were suspected as the diagnosis.

Warning: This exercise is not a means of diagnosing your headaches. The exercise is provided only to encourage you to carefully consider the features of your own headaches using a characterization of muscle contraction headaches for comparison. An accurate diagnosis of your headache problem requires a thorough medical evaluation by a trained professional. There is no acceptable substitute.

Profile
You have frequent headaches that are often present when you awake in the morning but may begin during the day. Usually they are not associated with visual symptoms or warning signs. They frequently hurt you in the forehead and the back of the head and

in the neck. You often feel as though a tight vise is squeezing your head and neck. The pain is not usually severe, as it can be in migraine. Heat applied to the back of the neck may make your headaches improve somewhat. Massage of your neck muscles seems to be helpful. Sleep is usually not disturbed by your attacks. Your headaches may last for days without any relief except when you sleep. You may be a nervous person or experience intense emotions, like anger and frustration. Perhaps you are depressed and tearful much of the time. You prefer to keep these feelings inside you. You may have arthritis of your neck or have suffered a previous injury to it. You take analgesics daily.

If this brief and general description of many muscle contraction headaches is similar to your headaches, you may want to answer the following questions. The questions are typical of some of those that would be asked of you if your physician suspected a diagnosis of muscle contraction headaches.

	True	False
1. Your headaches frequently begin soon after awakening in the morning but do not usually awaken you from sleep during the night.	——	——
2. Your neck and shoulders frequently hurt as part of your headaches.	——	——
3. Your headaches most commonly involve both sides of your neck and/or head.	——	——
4. Nausea and vomiting or distinct visual abnormalities are not typically present during your attacks.	——	——
5. Weakness, numbness, tingling, or other "neurological abnormalities" are not part of your headaches.	——	——
6. Warmth applied to your neck and head often brings you some relief.	——	——
7. Your headaches frequently feel as though a vise or handcuffs are squeezing your head.	——	——
8. Between your attacks you are in otherwise normal health.	——	——

True False

9. You are a nervous person and feel angry at many people and events but cannot seem to express yourself openly. ⸺ ⸺

10. Relaxing can often relieve your headaches. ⸺ ⸺

11. Maintaining certain postures of your neck and head for long periods, such as when typing, driving, or reading, can bring on a headache. ⸺ ⸺

12. Your headaches frequently last all day or until you go to sleep, only to return upon awaking in the morning. ⸺ ⸺

13. You often find yourself trying to "beat the clock" to finish a day's work and get things done. ⸺ ⸺

14. If you place a pillow under your neck so that your neck is bent backward slightly, your headaches seem to lessen. ⸺ ⸺

15. When you have a headache, you prefer to be active and occupy yourself rather than to lie quietly. ⸺ ⸺

16. You sometimes feel "knots" of tightened muscle in the back of your head or neck during a headache. ⸺ ⸺

17. You often feel depressed. ⸺ ⸺

18. Generally, your pain is only mildly to moderately intense, rather than severe. ⸺ ⸺

The characterization that you have just read and the questions that have been asked represent a profile of many muscle contraction headaches. If your headaches are similar to this presentation, please read carefully the following discussion about muscle contraction headaches.

THE MUSCLE CONTRACTION (TENSION) HEADACHE

"We'll be late!"
"The car won't start."
"What! He's done it again!"

"No, Mother, I'd rather do it myself."
"I have twelve chapters to read!"
"I hate going to work every day."
"I'm so angry at my boss that I could explode!"

Do your headaches have a tendency to occur when you are under emotional stress? If they do, it is likely that you have concluded that you have "tension headaches." But like other headaches, the condition called tension, or muscle contraction, headaches is terribly misunderstood, and the simple association between your headaches and stress does not alone qualify them for such a diagnosis. Many illnesses are provoked or worsened by emotional circumstances, and headaches of many types are triggered by stress, depression, and frustration.

Tension headache probably affects more people than any other type of headache. It is quite likely that the majority of day-to-day mild headaches, the kind that usually respond to a few aspirin, are due to muscle contraction. Most examples of this type of headache are so mild and easily treated with simple nonprescription analgesics that medical care is seldom sought. Our discussion will emphasize those muscle contraction headaches that are particularly persistent and unresponsive to simple analgesic therapy.

One factor that probably accounts for much of the misunderstanding that surrounds this disorder is the word "tension." The word "tension" in "tension headache" does not refer to emotional tension at all, but to tension, or spasm, of muscle. To avoid the obvious confusion, we will refer to this type of headache as a *muscle contraction headache,* since the origin of pain in this condition comes from spasms, or contractions, of neck, face, and scalp muscles. While emotional factors, like tension, anxiety, and worry, can provoke these spasms, they are not the only events that can trigger this painful condition. In some examples of this disorder, emotional stress is absent.

In order to understand this muscle contraction headache better, it should be recalled that the skull rests on a column of bones called vertebrae. Like other bones, the vertebrae of the spine and neck are held in position by tendons, ligaments, and many layers of muscle. The muscles surrounding the vertebrae are called

paraspinal muscles because they are located on the side (para-) of
the vertebral spines. The spines of the vertebrae are the bony
bumps you feel when running a finger up and down the center
of your neck and back.

Paraspinal muscles in the region of the neck extend upward
to join the base of the skull, overlapping other muscles running
down the back of the neck and into the shoulders. These muscles
support the vertebrae and skull and help control the movement
of the head, neck, and shoulders.

The skull, forehead, and facial bones are also surrounded by
thin layers of muscle, and these assist in moving the face, forehead, eyelids, nose, jaw, mouth, and, in a few people, the ears.
Smiling, squinting, frowning, and the furrowing of your brow
require the use of these muscles.

These muscles and most other muscles of the body are part of
an elaborate fully automatic system of reflexes that help protect
you against injury. Muscles play a critical role in this system;
emotional as well as physical factors can trigger the automatic
response.

When you suddenly sense danger, for example, muscles cause
your pupils to dilate, your heart muscle increases its rate of
contraction, and the muscles in the walls of some blood vessels
loosen to allow more blood to flow into your muscles and brain;
your entire body automatically prepares to defend itself against
the danger with the use of muscles. These functions represent a
physical response to, in the case of sensing danger, an *emotional*
stimulus. Blushing when you are embarrassed or turning pale
when fearful are additional examples of physical responses to
emotional circumstances.

An automatic physical response can also occur as a result of a
physical stimulus. For example, when a bone is fractured, the
muscles around the injured bone will contract and "splint" the
fracture and prevent movement and further injury. A similar
response occurs when your appendix becomes swollen and inflamed, the condition called appendicitis. Abdominal muscles
will contract tightly, making the abdomen rigid and protecting
the organs inside the body.

These automatic muscle responses are protective. But, unfortunately, the contraction of some muscles, like those around the head, neck, and back, also produces pain. While the pain serves to protect by way of warning of possible injury and preventing the movement of injured joints, which might be harmful, very often the pain of the muscle contraction is more intense than the injury or the situation that caused the muscles to react.

Keep in mind that the muscles around the head and neck cannot discern between emotional pain and physical distress, and a "splinting" protective response may occur when either emotional or physical assault is perceived in the head and neck region.

SYMPTOMS OF MUSCLE CONTRACTION HEADACHE

A muscle contraction headache is often described as a tight, squeezing, vise-like pain around the back of the head, the neck, the scalp, or the forehead. The entire face sometimes becomes painful. The discomfort can be like a band or rope of tightness or pressure around the head and neck. Some patients describe the pain as similar to that of wearing a hat many sizes too small.

The constant pain is usually dull, but sharp and jabbing knife-like pains about the head and neck can also occur. Muscle contraction headaches most often hurt on both sides, but one-sided headaches are not uncommon. The pain may spread down the shoulders and back, into the jaw, or behind the ears.

Muscle contraction headaches may begin at any time of the day, although they rarely awake their victims during the night. The morning is the most common time for the onset of an attack, but afternoon headaches are also frequent. If you are depressed and awaken early in the morning, a feature common to many depressed individuals, the pain may begin soon after.

A muscle contraction headache can last for a few hours, a few days, or even a few weeks. Unlike migraine, which often forces its victims into a dark room to sleep, many people with muscle contraction headache attempt to actively preoccupy themselves during painful experiences and often keep to their regular schedule, suffering in silence. Sleep is not usually disrupted by a muscle contraction headache, but many people awaken in the morning with the same headache that they had when they retired the night before.

A migraine headache is often preceded or accompanied by many additional symptoms, but aside from pain, there are few additional symptoms associated with muscle contraction headache. Nausea and vomiting and blurred vision may occur periodically. The headache does not have a distinguishable warning or pre-headache phase as does migraine, but many people who are troubled with muscle contraction headaches are also afflicted with migraine. A migraine headache or migraine-like throbbing pain may actually accompany muscle contraction headache, frequently subjecting the victim to double agony.

There is no clearcut relationship between the muscle contraction headache and foods, medications, or hormonal changes, as there is in migraine. Muscle contraction headaches do not seem to be an inherited problem, but usually more than one member of the family suffers from them. In other words, the tendency for the muscles around the head and neck to contract in an exaggerated way *may* also be biologically programmed, just as is the case in migraine. While genetic studies do not demonstrate a hereditary pattern, biological programming may have set an individual's "thermostat" in such a way that this reflex occurs more readily in some people than in others.

Muscle contraction headaches usually begin during adult life, although 10 to 20 percent of the victims may experience their first headaches in childhood or adolescence. Men and women seem to be more equally affected by muscle contraction headaches than in the case of migraine, which afflicts many more women than men.

WHY DO THE MUSCLES HURT?

Much of the pain associated with muscle contraction headaches comes from painfully contracted muscles, and this contraction can occasionally be felt by touching the scalp or neck muscles with your hand. The contracted muscles are often tender to any pressure and may feel like knots beneath the skin. Occasionally this tightness is evidenced by a furrowing of the brow or by a frown.

In addition to the muscle contraction, which in many ways is similar to a cramp, other abnormalities in the tissues, blood vessels, and tendons can add to the discomfort of this condition. In contrast to the vasodilation of migraine pain (an enlargement of the blood vessels), there is usually a constriction of blood vessels in muscle contraction headaches. Periodically, the blood vessels may dilate and throb. Medical science does not have a complete understanding of this process, but it seems likely that contracted muscles, a reduced blood supply, and an irritating substance found in the region of the pain are all responsible in a complicated way for the production of the discomfort.

WHAT TRIGGERS THE SPASM?

The following are only some of the events that can trigger muscle contraction headaches. Many of these headaches happen without any recognizable provoking factor.

Emotion—Prolonged worry, fear, depression, or internalized anger are all capable of causing the muscle contraction headache. A number of years ago, Dr. John R. Graham of Boston, a noted headache expert, compared the action of neck, scalp, and head muscles during emotionally disturbing events in humans and certain instinctive and automatic reflexes in animals threatened with danger. The neck and head muscles in the turtle, for example, automatically retract and pull the head under the protective cover of the shell. The ape also retracts its head into the well of the surrounding shoulders as the beast assumes the fighting posture. The similarity between this automatic response of lower animals and the automatic contraction of head and neck muscles in the human under stress raises the very interesting possibility that the automatic contraction of human neck and head muscles during emotional distress or danger represents a remnant of an automatic protective response in lower animals. In other words, the muscles of the head and neck contract in the presence of pain of the mind, just as the muscles of the arm respond to pain of a broken bone. Perhaps the body is trying to pull the head under a shell that does not exist, and in a skeleton composed of bones that cannot retract, as is the case with the lower animals. When we tell some of our patients that if they were turtles their head would be under the shell all or most of the time, they laugh approvingly, acknowledging their distress and the imagined relief at having some place to hide.

We know that stress, frustration, and depression are common elements in the personality of those who suffer from muscle contraction headaches, even though the presence of these strong feelings may not be recognized on a conscious level. You might ask yourself if your expression is always very serious, or if you have a frown on your face even when relaxing. Do you often clench your fists or jaw, perspire without apparent cause, gnash your teeth, or frequently seem worried or preoccupied with one problem or another? Do you have a hard time relaxing? Do you continually find fault with people and events around you? Do you have a problem relating to your mother or father, husband, wife, or partner? Do you feel anger for these people on the one hand and love on the other? Are you able to express these feelings openly or even accept them without guilt?

Your muscle contraction headaches may have no relationship to emotional stress. It is likely, however, that many sufferers from muscle contraction headaches do indeed trigger these headaches through a variety of emotional factors.

Some headache researchers believe that many muscle contraction headaches may occur in the morning hours because during sleep very emotionally distressful events come to the surface of our conscience. Jaw clenching, poor neck posture, and arthritis may also be important factors in provoking morning muscle contraction headaches. While sleep should be relaxing and restful, for many people with muscle contraction headaches sleeping is the most physically and emotionally distressful time of their day, because it is during this time that the mind expresses itself without restraint, and the body reacts appropriately.

Dr. Seymour Diamond of Chicago, a well-known headache authority, has coined the term "depression headache" to describe the morning headache affecting patients with continuing depression.

Disease of the Neck or Pain Elsewhere in the Body—Pain from abnormalities of the neck, eyes, teeth, jaw, or anywhere else in the body may incite muscle contraction of the head, neck, or face muscles.

Muscle contraction headaches frequently accompany cervical arthritis (arthritis of the neck). Arthritis is an inflammation of the joints, and this process may affect almost any joint in the body. There are many types of arthritis, but the two most common are called osteoarthritis (osteo- means bone) and rheumatoid arthritis. Rheumatoid arthritis is the most serious but fortunately the least common of the two. It is a disorder that may begin at any age and cause deformities of bone, frequently leading to crippling disabilities. Rheumatoid arthritis affects both young and old.

Osteoarthritis, also called degenerative arthritis, is by far the most common form of arthritis. This disorder eventually appears, to some extent, in almost everyone. It can affect nearly all joints of the body and is probably the result of years of physical stress on the joints. It can happen at any age but is most common after middle age. Most men and women over the age of forty-five show some evidence of osteoarthritis, but it can develop without apparent cause in younger people. Osteoarthritis causes pain on any movement of the involved joints, and it occasionally produces disability. When osteoarthritis affects the neck, the likelihood of developing muscle contraction headaches is increased. In part, this may be due to an automatic response of the muscles to "splint" the damaged bones against harmful movement, or the muscle contraction may be a response to the pain.

The arthritis can be severe or located in a critical spot. When this happens, portions of the degenerating bone can press on nerves and cause pain as well as neurological impairment. This process is referred to as a "pinched nerve" because the nerve becomes compressed, irritated, and subsequently inflamed. When the nerve is compressed, either by arthritis or by a vertebral disc (the "cushion" separating the vertebrae), pain, tingling, numbness, and weakness may develop. When the compression involves the nerves going to the arms or legs, the pains are often referred down the entire arm or leg. When the upper cervical nerves are involved, the pain from those nerves and the muscle contraction that is triggered by the pain may be referred up the back of the head.

Abnormalities of the neck, other than arthritis, can also trigger muscle contraction headaches. Injuries of the neck, such as whiplash, tumors of the spine, or congenital (present at birth) deformities of the vertebrae or skull may result in pain and associated muscle contraction, which causes even more pain.

It seems that when any disease of the neck is present, muscle contraction headaches may be more easily triggered by emotional events than if the abnormality in the neck did not exist. In other words, abnormal conditions of the structures around the head and neck make it more likely for muscles of that region to painfully contract as a result of emotional factors, or any other triggering influences for that matter.

As we have already suggested, it is not uncommon for people with migraine to occasionally experience muscle contraction headaches at the same time they are suffering from a severe migraine attack. Perhaps this is due to an unconscious attempt to hold the painful, throbbing head and neck immobile, since movement during the migraine attack is often nauseating and quite painful. Another explanation, however, is that pain from the migraine serves as a triggering stimulus for automatic muscle contraction.

Posture or Prolonged Use of Muscles—If you hold your head and neck rigid or in an awkward position for a long period of time, muscle pain may develop. This is common in persons who become tense while driving their automobiles in bad weather or heavy traffic. Bedtime television watchers may provoke this discomfort by slouching in bed with the head propped forward by a pillow as they peer at the television set located at the foot of the bed. Looking down while reading may also lead to muscle contraction pain. This chin-on-chest posture is apt to be particularly uncomfortable for anyone who has a preexisting arthritis in the neck. Prolonged extension of the neck upward and backward, as when painting a ceiling, can, of course, also be painful.

One of our patients noted that she suffered headaches only on the evenings that she played cards with friends. The headache would usually begin late in the evening, after she had spent many hours looking down at the cards she held in her hands. Concentrating on the cards and enduring the smoke in the room cannot be entirely overlooked as contributing factors, but it eventually became clear that the woman's chin-on-chest posture was to a large extent responsible for producing the discomfort. She was given a cervical collar to wear during her card parties. This device is worn around the neck and assists in supporting the head and limits the forward movement of the head and neck. To the patient's delight, and to ours as well, her headaches lessened, and the pain did not interfere with her enjoyment of the game.

The chin-on-chest posture often produces discomfort in those of you whose work or other activities require this position for long periods. Typing, reading, propping a telephone receiver between the shoulder and head while talking, and similar activities can cause headaches in some people.

Facial mannerisms, such as prolonged frowning, squinting, jaw clenching, gum chewing, teeth gnashing, even holding a smile or other movements of the face requiring specific muscle activity, may also provoke muscle pain that is felt as a headache. If you have arthritis of the jaw joint, imbalances, or other abnormalities of your jaw, the muscles around your jaw and temple area may painfully contract when the jaw is used, particularly during prolonged or intense chewing activity. This is often felt as a headache in the ear area or temple region.

DIAGNOSING THE MUSCLE CONTRACTION HEADACHE

The diagnosis of muscle contraction headache, like that of migraine, is based heavily on noting the characteristic special symptoms of the headache and finding out exactly what activates the headache's occurrence. A thorough physical examination is necessary, and during the examination, special attention must be given to the areas from which the pain seems to come. A careful manual search for sensitive points must be carried out. Cautious bending forward and bending backward, along with rotation of the head in a variety of positions, can sometimes point up the positions that provoke pain. Spasm and contraction of the neck muscles can occasionally be felt, but between attacks the muscles may feel normal.

X rays of the skull and neck are often performed to determine whether there is any evidence of bone abnormalities. The jaw and the jaw joint must be evaluated as well. The muscles, nerves, and spinal cord and other soft tissues cannot be evaluated effectively by routine X rays, which show only bone or tissue containing calcium. A manual examination of the head and neck should not be neglected simply because X rays are ordered.

Invasive diagnostic tests, the type that enter the body and cause risks, are generally not required unless important abnormalities are spotted during the X ray or the manual examinations. You and your doctor must recognize that the presence of muscle contraction means that there is a possibility that a specific disease is responsible for the contraction, and this must be considered in the evaluation.

Likewise, it is very important in some patients to look for relevant emotional distress. While many of our patients are offended if we raise the possibility, you should be receptive to a psychological interview to determine *if*, in fact, there are elements of anger, depression, rage, or other issues that are known to be present in many patients with muscle contraction headaches. It is our opinion that as long as your doctor shows an open-minded attitude towards *all* possible factors, not *just* emotional ones, you should not resist an inquiry into the emotional elements that could be important in creating your headache cycle.

TREATING THE MUSCLE CONTRACTION HEADACHE

The basic elements of treatment for muscle contraction headaches include reassurance, the establishment of a trusting relationship between the patient and the doctor, the removal of physical or emotional triggering factors, and treatment of the discomfort. This is not very different from what has been suggested as the treatment for migraine.

If a physical illness is present, that abnormality must be treated appropriately. If no physical abnormalities can be found to account for the headaches, it is often assumed that emotions play a critical role in the production of the headaches. This presumption should not be made prematurely, since emotional upset usually accompanies or follows any prolonged and painful event. Simply suffering from a regular and sometimes daily pain is enough to cause the "pain-distress" cycle in which pain triggers the emotional upset and the emotional upset triggers the pain. It is, therefore, very important not to simply assume that emotion is the cause of the muscle contraction headaches, even though features of emotional upset may be present.

To interrupt and stop the pain-distress cycle and to alleviate the pain, it is often necessary to use combinations of analgesics, muscle relaxants, tranquilizers, and antidepressants. The use of these medications, particularly analgesics and tranquilizers, must be temporary. Regular and continued use of many of these drugs is potentially harmful to your body. Prolonged use of drugs encourages the development of emotional as well as physical dependence.

There seems to be a strong tendency for patients with recurring muscle contraction headaches to abusively use pain-relieving and tranquilizing medication. Not only does this have physical consequences, such as injuring the stomach, liver, and kidneys, but this abuse actually promotes headaches and physical and emotional dependence on these agents. The antidepressants (see below) may be appropriate for somewhat longer periods of time in certain situations, but indefinite reliance on any medication, including these, must be considered a failure of the overall headache treatment program.

A wide variety of analgesics can be used to treat the *occasional* muscle contraction headache. Aspirin and acetaminophen (Tylenol and Datril) are relatively safe and often very helpful. Combination drugs are widely used although many doctors tend to avoid their use whenever possible.

Fiorinal is a combination brand-name drug, available in cheaper generic versions, that combines a barbiturate sedative, aspirin, phenacetin (a simple but potentially dangerous analgesic), and caffeine. Phenacetin, while an effective analgesic, can, like some other analgesics, injure the kidneys if there is prolonged and regular use. This combination product is popular and effective in many circumstances, but is so frequently abused that we generally discourage its use except occasionally.

In Canada, phenacetin has been removed from all combination drug products containing salicylates (such as aspirin). In the United States, phenacetin is still available in prescription drugs (not in over-the-counter products), but it is likely that phenacetin will soon be removed from such prescription drugs in the United States as well.

Norgesic is a combination drug that contains orphenadrine (a muscle relaxant), aspirin, phenacetin, and caffeine.

Parafon Forte is another combination medication combining the muscle relaxant chlorzoxazone and acetaminophen.

Propoxyphene (Darvon) is a very popular analgesic used for a variety of painful conditions. This drug is chemically related to narcotics, and abuse and dependence, as well as withdrawal problems, develop if the drug is used over a long period of time. Darvon comes in a plain form and in combination with a variety of simple analgesics, including aspirin, phenacetin, and acetaminophen.

Codeine is a narcotic analgesic that can be added to a large number of simple analgesics. It is a fairly effective and relatively safe pain reliever but abuse commonly occurs, although not to the extent observed with more potent narcotic analgesics.

For patients with frequently recurring muscle contraction headaches, antidepressants seem to be the most effective drugs. Scientific observations, such as those by Dr. Donald Dalessio, a noted headache expert from La Jolla, California, have shown that the antidepressants, such as amitriptyline (Endep and Elavil), may be quite helpful in treating this disorder. Other antidepressants of similar structure are also widely employed.

It is our opinion that for daily muscle contraction headaches these antidepressants are perhaps the most effective medications available. It is important to keep in mind that their benefit may have nothing to do with their effect as an antidepressant. In fact, patients who are not depressed will generally not experience any change in mood as a result of these drugs. Their benefit may be due to a mechanism that influences muscle contraction; drugs of similar structure are used as muscle relaxants. Additionally, there is some sparse evidence suggesting that these antidepressant medications may exert a primary effect on pain control centers and have been found useful in the treatment of diverse causes of chronic pain such as cancer, diabetes, and pain following certain types of infections.

It is not unusual in our experience for patients with daily pain to find themselves taking ten to twenty analgesic tablets each day, a quantity that is unquestionably hazardous to mind and body. Furthermore, relief of pain may require complete discontinuance of all analgesic medication, since, in a yet-to-be-defined way, regular use of analgesics may actually lower your pain threshold. It is often necessary to hospitalize patients to withdraw these medications safely and completely.

The preventive medications can be useful not only in providing some relief to the patient but also in helping to eliminate the harmful medications on which the patient may have become dependent. During this "plateau" of relief, it is important to work very hard to develop insight into the cause of the pain and to pursue non-medicinal interventions for long-term control.

It is for this and other reasons that recent research regarding biofeedback and muscle contraction is so important. A score of headache experts have shown impressive results using biofeedback and relaxation methods for treatment of recurring muscle contraction headaches. Dr. Lee Kudrow of Encino, California, one such headache authority, has actually found that patients undergoing biofeedback treatment for muscle contraction headaches who are able and willing to give up analgesics had better long-term results from the biofeedback treatment than patients who continued to use pain relievers along with the biofeedback therapy. Biofeedback is becoming the treatment of choice for muscle contraction headaches, particularly in young people.

We have found that, in addition to biofeedback and the cautious use of some medications, cervical collars for support and the maintenance of good posture, neck traction, and careful exercise of the neck muscles may be an effective way to treat many people.

The application of heat, regular massage, perhaps using a vibrator, and formal physical therapy can be very successful. Sleeping on a pillow that supports the neck and allows a slightly backward posture of the head may prove beneficial for some patients.

When emotional factors are crucial in the production of muscle contraction headaches, a trusting relationship with your physician is essential. The doctor must assist you to modify the circumstances in your life that may provoke your headaches. Muscle contraction headaches often develop or worsen at the same time that emotional burdens intensify.

It is essential to once again stress that if your doctor asks you to undergo a psychological evaluation to help identify areas of anger or hostility, to help modify certain situations in your life, to help you learn to express your feelings more openly, deal with stress less harmfully, or learn to relax, you should not resist or resent such recommendations. Those of us who see many patients in pain, particularly with muscle contraction headaches, have come to recognize, through many years of experience, that these interventions may play a dramatically effective role in bringing relief and a healthier life.

Chronic unrelenting stress must be recognized as a serious health hazard, and any legitimate effort to relieve it should be considered beneficial and wholesome.

An active, productive, and useful life, together with a feeling of self-reliance, is also beneficial. Good eating habits, regular exercise, adequate rest, and learning to relax and enjoy life's pleasures are all important in the total headache treatment. This may mean restructuring the pattern of your life, or it may require only minimal but crucial modifications. In the end, your active participation in your own therapy, together with the advice and counseling of a concerned physician, is the essential ingredient in treating this troublesome headache disorder.

During the past several years, headache authorities have come to recognize that the mechanism of most chronic headaches, particularly those suffered daily, have both muscle contraction *and* vascular components. The history is characterized by daily occurring muscle contraction pain and periodic migraine or migraine-like headaches, approximately once every week or so. Many patients suffering from this disorder take excessive amounts of analgesics. Successful treatment often requires therapy directed at both muscular and vascular elements. Often nonmedicinal interventions such as biofeedback and psychotherapy may be necessary in addition to appropriate medications.

Chapter 4 Cluster Headaches

THE CLUSTER HEADACHE PROFILE

The Cluster Headache Profile below is a description of the symptoms of cluster headaches. It is followed by a series of questions that a physician might ask you if cluster headaches were suspected as the diagnosis.

Warning: This exercise is not a means of diagnosing your headaches. The exercise is provided only to encourage you to carefully consider the features of your own headaches using a characterization of cluster headaches for comparison. An accurate diagnosis of your headache problem requires a thorough evaluation by a trained professional. There is no acceptable substitute.

Profile

You have recurring headaches on one side of your face; your eye and jaw on that side are also involved. The headaches occur in episodes lasting fifteen minutes to an hour each. The attacks can occur one to six times during the day and night and tend to repeat in bouts that last for weeks or months. You may go for months or even years without a recurrence.

During an attack, you may experience, on the affected side of your face, a runny nose, tearing, and a bloodshot eye. You do not have a warning that an attack will occur. Your attacks often come during the nighttime, awakening you from a sound sleep one or more times. The pain is excruciating. Ingestion of any form of alcoholic beverage almost invariably brings on an attack during one of the bouts.

If this brief and general description of cluster headaches is similar to your headaches, you may want to answer the following questions. The questions are typical of some of those that would be asked of you if your physician suspected a diagnosis of cluster headaches.

	True	False
1. Your headaches began after the age of twenty.	——	——
2. Your attacks occur in groups, or clusters, of at least one to six per day.	——	——
3. Each bout of headaches lasts for one to three months at a time.	——	——
4. A headache can be brought on by drinking alcohol during a bout of attacks.	——	——
5. Between attacks, you are in good health.	——	——
6. You are without headaches most of the time except for the cluster period.	——	——
7. Your headaches are worsened by bending over.	——	——
8. During an attack, your nose, on the same side as the pain, is runny.	——	——
9. During an attack, your eye, on the side of the headache, tears or waters.	——	——
10. You feel like pacing, running, screaming, or thrusting your fist or head against a wall during a headache.	——	——
11. You are a heavy smoker.	——	——
12. You are inclined to drink alcohol frequently.	——	——

The characterization that you have just read and the questions that have been asked represent a profile of many cluster headaches. If your headaches are similar to this presentation, please read carefully the following discussion about cluster headaches.

THE CLUSTER HEADACHE

We have been using the term "vascular headaches" to refer to a group of headache conditions that share the common feature of having blood vessel widening as a major component in the production of painful symptoms. Migraine is the best-known headache disorder of this group. Another headache of this vascular headache group is a condition called cluster headache. This headache claims the notorious distinction of being one of the most painful conditions known to medical science. So ravaging is this headache that suicide has not only been contemplated but carried out as a means of escaping the agony of this affliction.

Cluster headaches are known by a variety of names. They are also called histamine headaches because this chemical is perhaps related to the sequence of events in this syndrome. Histamine, you may recall, is one of the amine substances that play an important role in causing the pain and inflammation associated with allergic conditions.

Sometimes cluster headaches are called Horton's headaches, after the physician who first described this condition in the United States. Cluster headaches have also been referred to as "red headaches" because of the heat and flushing of the face that sometimes accompany the attacks. This coloring contrasts with the pallor that often accompanies a migraine headache.

Two other terms for this disorder are "episodic migrainous neuralgia" and "Harris' neuralgia." "Harris' neuralgia" is the term used in some parts of Europe and refers to Dr. Wilfred Harris, an English neurologist who first described the disorder. We use the term "cluster headaches" because it emphasizes the characteristic grouping of attacks. Each cluster, or group, of headaches may last several weeks or even months at a time before either suddenly or gradually fading away for months or years.

Cluster headaches afflict more men than women. The reverse

is true in migraine. Migraine frequently begins early in life; cluster headaches do not usually begin before the age of twenty-five, and most commonly the onset of these painful headaches occurs after the age of thirty. The exact cause of cluster headache is not known, but this should not come as any great surprise since this is true with many other headache conditions as well. Although vasodilation and some other chemical changes do occur during a cluster attack, the reasons for the repetitive tendency of cluster headaches, for the excruciating intensity of pain, and for the periodic nature of the bouts remain medical mysteries.

SYMPTOMS OF CLUSTER HEADACHE

Cluster headaches usually develop without warning. There is a tendency for the attacks to occur at specific times of the day or night, often with such regularity that some of our patients claim that they can actually set their watches by the onset of the pain. The repetitive episodes are quite uniform and vary only slightly from attack to attack. Typically, the attacks recur one to six times each twenty-four hours, frequently awakening their victims from a sound sleep a few hours after retiring.

The pain of a cluster headache can be overwhelming. It almost always begins on one side of the upper face or head, often near one eye, the forehead, or the temple. The pain then spreads to other areas on the same side of the face or head. As the intensity of the pain grows, it usually localizes around or in an eye or over one temple. The pain is present on only one side of the face and neck at a time but may alternate, affecting the other side in separate attacks.

During an attack, the nose on the painful side of the face often becomes stuffy or runny. The eye on the affected side may become bloodshot and tears may run copiously down the side of the face. Occasionally, the eyelid will droop, the pupil on the affected side will narrow, and the skin of the involved side of the face may become warm and flushed. Despite the severity of the pain, nausea and vomiting do not regularly occur.

The intensity of the pain of a cluster headache deserves special mention. It has been described as

burning,
throbbing,
boring,
piercing,
tearing, or
stabbing.

It usually begins as a mild but distinct discomfort, then quickly, over a period of minutes, relentlessly gathers intensity. The pain can be incredibly cruel and merciless, and those who suffer from it vividly attest to its excruciating torture.

Cluster headaches have been described as the most painful event imaginable. One of our patients described each attack as feeling as though a red-hot iron were being pressed into his forehead and eye until it had burned its way through his skull. Another said of his attacks that they felt as though the skin of his face and his eyes were being clawed from his skull and acid poured into the open wound. Another victim described the attacks as a burning metal spike being pounded into his eye and pushed through the skull, deep into his brain. One patient likened his attacks to the flame of a blowtorch being applied to his eye for fifteen to twenty minutes. It is not unusual for people who are normally stoic to scream out in anguish during an attack.

During a migraine attack, darkness and quiet are often sought, but individuals who suffer with cluster headaches often desperately pace, sometimes banging their heads against walls or inflicting painful bodily injury to themselves in order to alter the feeling of head pain.

Not long ago, the wife of a patient with cluster headaches phoned at five o'clock in the morning. She was sobbing and panic-stricken. In the background could be heard her husband's loud and agonized screaming. The woman was crying and asking whether she should take her husband to the hospital. As she spoke, a loud banging sound became audible over the telephone, and the woman said that it was her husband banging his head on a tabletop; he threatened to commit suicide unless he could escape from the searing pain.

Each attack of cluster headache lasts from fifteen minutes to an hour, averaging about thirty minutes. To most victims the period seems forever. The attack can subside suddenly or gradually, but a dull ache may last for a while afterward. The individual is then well until another attack strikes.

Drinking alcoholic beverages is likely to provoke some migraine attacks, but alcohol's ability to initiate a cluster episode is dramatic. Most people with cluster headaches are exquisitely sensitive to alcohol, particularly during a bout of headaches. Strangely, however, alcohol may not trigger an attack during the headache-free months. One of our patients said that during his cluster attacks even the smell of a strong alcoholic drink would make him sick with a headache, but he could drink without restraint during his headache-free intervals.

Cluster headaches occur more commonly during the spring and fall, but can develop during any season. With some patients, years will pass between attacks. Every so often a victim will experience attacks that do not cluster but will continue year after year without remission. In other words, the cluster headaches just do not cluster. (What's in a name anyway!)

While cluster headache is generally a condition that occurs in bouts, there is a form of it called *chronic cluster headaches,* in which the attacks do not have a merciful period of remission. Patients experience attacks every day, often numerous times per day, and these attacks may go on for years at a time without remission. Dr. Ninan Mathew of Houston, Texas, and Dr. Lee Kudrow of Encino, California, both well-known cluster headache experts, have helped us understand more completely this chronic headache entity, as well as the classic cluster headache.

One of our patients came to us after ten years of at least five attacks a day. He claimed that throughout the entire period he had enjoyed only two months during which he did not suffer from his headaches. He told us that if he could not find relief soon he was going to end his life. We are still working with this patient, and although he is dramatically improved, he still endures an occasional headache every few months.

While cluster attacks usually bear a striking similarity from one patient to another, some people do have attacks that deviate from the classical pattern. Instead of being localized mainly around an eye or temple, the pain may center around the lower part of the face, the upper or lower cheek, the jaw, and even the neck. This variation has been called a "lower-half headache" and may be easily confused with the pain of dental origin. There is some difference of opinion among medical experts about these lower-face attacks with respect to whether they are related to typical cluster headaches or not.

SOME INTERESTING CHARACTERISTICS OF CLUSTER HEADACHE SUFFERERS

Interesting similarities among the victims of cluster headaches have been observed. For years Dr. John R. Graham, a cluster headache authority, has recognized that many cluster headache patients have a rugged facial appearance, with coarse, wrinkled, and highly textured skin. Recently, Dr. Lee Kudrow studied physical characteristics of a large group of cluster patients and produced a number of interesting findings. Men with cluster headaches tend to be taller than average and frequently have blue or hazel-colored eyes. They have a greater than average tendency to have thicker blood (high hemoglobin) than those who do not suffer from cluster headaches. Another very interesting finding was that 94 percent of cluster headache victims smoked cigarettes, compared to only 63 percent in the non-cluster-headache population. People with cluster headaches smoked an average of thirty-two cigarettes a day, while the control group (the group that did not have cluster headaches) averaged only twenty-one per day. And another intriguing observation was that despite the known sensitivity to alcohol during the cluster period, a striking 91 percent of cluster patients drank strong alcoholic beverages and almost two-thirds of the victims considered themselves heavy drinkers. This contrasts strikingly with the control group, in which only 65 percent were drinkers and only 20 percent of that group considered themselves heavy drinkers.

Furthermore, there seems to be depressive tendencies in some patients with cluster headaches. It is not unusual for patients to experience not only depressive-type symptoms, but also sleep disturbances (common in depression) during their cluster bouts. These observations are intriguing, but the exact meaning of the data remains uncertain.

HOW CLUSTER HEADACHE IS DIAGNOSED

The diagnosis of cluster headache is usually established through a medical history that notes the characteristic features of the attacks, and by eliminating other conditions that can be confused with or that simulate the disorder. Despite the distinct and classical features of this headache syndrome, the diagnosis of cluster headache is sometimes overlooked, and dental problems, allergies, and even inflamed sinuses are cited as the cause for the pain. Before the diagnosis of cluster headache has been correctly established, some cluster headache sufferers have undergone surgery on their nasal septums or have endured tooth extractions, all to no avail.

WHAT TRIGGERS CLUSTER HEADACHE?

Emotional triggering of a headache is common in migraine and, of course, in muscle contraction headaches, but emotion does not appear to have the same importance in triggering a cluster headache. Many of our patients do suffer significant emotional upset, but often this reflects the devastating impact of the condition itself. The horrible pain often makes the victims behave in bizarre and unusual ways, and thus appear unstable.

We have already mentioned that alcoholic drinks can trigger a cluster headache. Some attacks are provoked by smoking or by being in smoke-filled rooms. Exertion or exercise can also provoke an attack. Recently a thirty-five-year-old truck driver came to us. He had been suffering three to four cluster attacks a day without remission for almost four years. The attacks tended to be the same whether he was on the road or at home between hauls. In order to isolate any triggering event and to try various therapies, he was admitted to the hospital for observation. During the first week in the hospital, the patient did not have even one attack, despite our attempts to provoke them. It was not until the man once again began his morning ritual of exercises, which he had not done during the first week in the hospital, that his attacks recurred. In retrospect, he realized that it was days on which he unloaded his haul that his attacks were invariably worse. When he was at home, he did morning exercises, as well as some heavy work, which was likewise physically exerting. The patient has since tried to restrict this physical stress. With the use of medications and these minor modifications, his attacks have lessened considerably and he only occasionally suffers headaches.

Many other factors can trigger cluster headaches. Drugs or foods that dilate blood vessels, like the nitrite-containing substances in hot dogs or smoked meats, can provoke an attack. Some people find that rapidly changing temperature, like a sudden cold or hot wind in the face, will trigger a headache.

THE TREATMENT OF CLUSTER HEADACHE

Successful treatment of cluster headaches is often difficult. Each attack usually lasts for less than an hour, so by the time medication taken by mouth is absorbed into the bloodstream, the attack has already run its course. The ergotamines are sometimes effective if taken at the onset of an attack by a way that gets the drug into the bloodstream rapidly, such as a rectal suppository, a lozenge held under the tongue, or by the inhalant form of the medication.

Sometimes the ergotamines are taken two or three times a day to prevent the attacks. Extreme caution must be observed, because ergotamine should not be used this frequently, since these medications may have serious side effects when taken daily, particularly for any extended length of time. But because the attacks are so painful, and if it appears that only the ergotamines will relieve the discomfort, these drugs are nevertheless reluctantly administered daily. This therapy must be carried out under careful medical supervision, and for brief periods only. If the siege of headaches continues for a long time, ergotamines are not suitable.

Another drug frequently successful for cluster headache is methysergide (Sansert), which, like the ergotamines, has potentially serious side effects (see page 85). Methysergide is given daily to prevent the attacks but is potentially hazardous when used without interruption for more than six months at a time. Since a cluster attack usually lasts for only a few weeks or a month or two, methysergide therapy can be used without undue risk, although we use it only when less potentially hazardous medications fail to bring relief.

Propranolol (Inderal; see page 84) has recently been shown to help some cluster headache patients, and this drug does not seem to possess the risks associated with methysergide therapy. Both propranolol and methysergide are designed to be taken daily to prevent the headaches rather than to treat them once an attack occurs.

Recently, a major breakthrough in the treatment of cluster headaches has been achieved. Drs. Kudrow and Mathew, using preliminary information from work by Dr. Karl Ekbom, have shown that certain patients with cluster headaches, particularly those whose headaches do not cluster but are continuous without remissions (chronic), may respond to the drug lithium. Lithium has been used for years to treat emotionally disturbed patients who suffer from major and inappropriate swings in their mood, ranging from severe depression to mania (overactivity and hyperexcitability).

Exactly how lithium works on either manic-depressive disease or cluster headaches is not known, but considering Drs. Kudrow and Mathew and our use of this drug, it does appear that lithium may be of real value in treating many cluster headache patients who have thus far been without successful treatment.

Lithium should not be taken without careful monitoring of blood levels. When a person is taking lithium, it is appropriate for the physician to order lithium blood levels at regular intervals in order to avoid overmedication with this substance. Lithium may have toxic side effects on the thyroid and the kidney. In addition, the level of lithium in the bloodstream can be influenced by certain dietary substances. Ingesting large amounts of salty food, for example, may reduce the effectiveness of lithium. Dietary restriction of salt (sodium chloride) or the simultaneous use of water pills (diuretics), which cause the body to lose salt, may cause the lithium in the bloodstream to rise and have a toxic effect. Many authorities believe that lithium can be used at low dosages reasonably safely, as long as careful monitoring and instruction take place. Nevertheless, some toxic effects of lithium have been reported even at low doses. You should not take this drug without proper instruction and careful monitoring.

Cortisone-like drugs (steroids) can be successful in the treatment of cluster headaches, particularly when the attacks do not respond to other medications. Cortisone drugs are potentially harmful when use is sustained, and they should not customarily be used for prolonged periods of time for cluster headaches. Some individuals will get relief by breathing pure oxygen (constricts blood vessels) when a cluster attack is just beginning, and this therapy has sometimes brought dramatic results. Cyproheptadine (Periactin; see page 84) may at times be helpful.

Because sensitivity to histamine has for a long time been considered one of the villains that cause cluster headaches, reduction of the body's sensitivity to this amine has been undertaken in an attempt to prevent the recurrence of attacks. This desensitization process is carried out by administering small injections of histamine over a period of weeks in order to lessen the body's responsiveness to histamine's effects. Although this therapy is recommended by some headache investigators, our experience is that histamine desensitization is only occasionally successful in the prevention of cluster headaches, and we are not at all certain that it is valuable in the treatment of most cluster headaches.

Recently, chlorpromazine (Thorazine) and related drugs have shown promise in helping some patients with cluster headaches.

As in other headache conditions, no single therapy is successful in treating every case. After initial success with one or more drugs, some people break through their therapy and the drugs are no longer effective; in these cases, other treatments must be found. Abstinence from alcohol and tobacco, as well as trying to eliminate other triggering factors, is, of course, very important. One of the remarkable ironies associated with this condition is that despite the devastating impact of the pain, many persons who suffer from cluster headaches continue to drink and smoke heavily, apparently choosing to rely on medicine to overcome the triggering effect of these activities.

While there are a few patients who continue to suffer attacks despite treatment, most people with cluster headaches can be helped. After a number of years of recurrence with or without successful treatment, the headaches will gradually subside in intensity and frequency and will finally be gone.

The following is a case report of a patient with cluster headaches.

A 30-year-old graduate student had been in good health for his entire life. A friendly and sociable type, he enjoyed going out on Saturday evenings to drink with his friends. On the evening that his attacks first began, the student had consumed only half a stein of beer when he suddenly developed a burning pain over his right temple and eye. Within a few minutes the pain became excruciating and the student was screaming in agony.

His alarmed friends noticed that his right eye was tearing, bloodshot, and the lid was drooping. In desperation, the student began to pound his head with his clenched fist. His friends, fearing that he had ruptured a blood vessel, called an ambulance. By the time the ambulance arrived, the attack had subsided and the student refused to go to the hospital. He went home and to bed.

During the night, the student awoke with a second attack identical to the first. This one lasted thirty minutes. By morning, he felt better and so did not seek medical attention. During the next two or three days, he continued to suffer three or four attacks per day, sometimes being awakened at 2:00 A.M. or 4:00 A.M. in agony. Finally, the student went to a drugstore and bought a sinus headache medicine, reasoning that because of the runny nose and the tearing eye, along with pain over an eye, a sinus infection was a likely explanation for the fierce headaches.

After experiencing no relief from the sinus headache medication, the student sought the assistance of a dentist. He was examined and was told that a few bad teeth might be responsible for his pain. He had the cavities filled. Although the student continued to suffer from the attacks for a week after that, they gradually lessened in intensity and frequency, eventually fading away.

Approximately eight months later the attacks recurred. They were identical to the earlier headaches and came four to five times a day. The student went back to the dentist, who told him that he did not think that the problem was due to the student's teeth and suggested that he see a general physician.

The student followed this advice, and a physician told him that he believed the recurring headaches were due to a deviated nasal septum and suggested surgery. Seeking another opinion, the student consulted a second physician who made the diagnosis of cluster headaches.

The student was placed on a combination of medications that dramatically reduced the intensity and frequency of the attacks. Since that time, the patient has utilized these medications whenever the attacks recur, averaging about two to three clusters per year.

Recently, a series of medical reports have described a condition strikingly similar to cluster headaches but which occurs in young women. This disorder is called chronic paroxysmal hemicrania. Although similar in many ways to cluster headaches, chronic paroxysmal hemicrania characteristically improves with the drug Indocin (indomethacin), traditionally used to treat arthritis.

Chapter 5 Sinus Headaches, or Madison Avenue's "Gift" to Medicine

So you think that you have sinus headaches. The pain is over your eyes, forehead, or bridge of your nose. The discomfort is throbbing, as though hammers were pounding away at your head. There is pressure in your eyes and around your forehead, just as if little "drains" were blocked. Nasal stuffiness or discharge and tearing eyes sometimes accompany your pain. Perhaps the pain is worse when low-pressure weather fronts move into your vicinity or when you bend over.

Who would challenge the similarity between your headache symptoms and the illustrative advertisements that so generously offer you free medical instruction and advice? The truth is that most of you who believe that you have sinus headaches probably suffer from migraine or other chronic headache condition not at all related to disease of your sinuses.

Rarely does the day pass that a number of patients with recurring headaches do not state that they are victims of sinus headache, believing that sinus trouble accounts for their distress. When questioned, they suggest that their headaches are identical to those depicted in the sinus headache commercials on television.

It is estimated that more than 80 percent of individuals who suffer from recurring headaches have at one time or another bought and tried various sinus headache remedies. Nevertheless, by our estimates and those of many specialists in eye, ear, nose, and throat diseases, who are experts in disease of sinuses, only one of every fifty people seeking help for "sinus trouble" actually suffers from sinus disease.

This widespread misunderstanding requires clarification. Within the layers of bone forming the skull are numerous spaces called sinuses, which are lined by sensitive tissue—the mucous membranes. Sinuses are present on either side of the nose and in the forehead. The tissue lining the sinuses is endowed with many blood vessels, and its nerve supply is via branches of the fifth cranial nerve, the trigeminal nerve.

The tissue in the sinuses secretes mucus, and this fluid must have a means of draining out of the sinuses. This is accomplished through small openings in the floor of the sinuses, openings that empty into the nose. Understandably, any disturbance that blocks the passage of fluid out of the sinuses will soon cause a backup of fluid and a buildup of pressure. From this will come pain.

A number of abnormal processes can block the outflow drains. Infection in the sinuses causes inflammation of the tissue lining, and this, together with swelling and dilation of the many blood vessels located in the sinus tissue, will produce a blockage. Acute allergic reactions can produce inflammation, swelling, and blockage as well. Tumors in the sinuses can also produce similar symptoms.

No one would argue that these conditions could cause sinus symptoms and headaches. One source of the misunderstanding is that migraine and other vascular headache entities can also cause many of the same symptoms. During a migraine attack, the blood vessels around the head and face become dilated, and this dilation can involve the blood vessels of the sinus tissue as well. This enlargement makes the discomfort of migraine similar to that of infectious and allergic sinus headaches. The typical features of cluster headaches, for example, include tearing eyes, runny or stuffy nose, and pain in the forehead, face, and eyes. Many migraines do the same.

Another important cause of the misunderstanding is the almost universal association of head pain and weather changes. As you may recall from earlier discussions in the migraine chapter, it has been shown that when the weather changes, many patients will experience a variety of physiological symptoms, among which may be headache. Some researchers suggest that this is due to changes in air ions that accompany low-pressure weather fronts. They speculate that the ions have an effect on body chemistry that can influence changes in body function. Television commercials advertising sinus headache remedies frequently associate bad weather with sinus pain, misleading the public to believe that bad weather and headaches generally mean sinus discomfort.

The point, of course, is that migraine and the other vascular headaches affect an estimated twenty million people in this country. Sinus disease affects many fewer people. Both can cause similar symptoms. Additionally, pain anywhere along the fifth cranial nerve° can be referred to the area around the sinuses, mimicking pain coming from the sinuses.

Having said all of this, it must now be emphasized that there is such a condition as the sinus headache. When it is present, most of the symptoms that we have described occur. But when disease of the sinuses is causing the headache, there will very often be fever if infection is present, allergic symptoms if acute allergic reaction is present, and, importantly, X rays of the sinuses will usually show that blockage has occurred. The features required to establish the diagnosis of sinus disease are usually not present in most people who think that they are suffering from sinus headache. The reason is that there is nothing primarily wrong with their sinuses.

Why then, if sinus headaches are relatively rare, are the sinus headache remedies so popular? It is our opinion that this is so for two reasons. First, all of the sinus headache remedies contain either or both aspirin or acetaminophen, and these substances

° See Appendix.

should lessen some muscle contraction headaches and even some migraine masquerading as sinus headaches. Secondly, we believe people are so convinced that they have sinus disease that when they take a highly advertised sinus headache remedy, a placebo response may well be of some assistance in the initial pain relief. Actually, most people state that the sinus headache remedies only dull their headaches and do not take them away altogether. This could well be explained by the mild analgesic effect of the aspirin or acetaminophen.

Most people who have headaches that involve the forehead, eyes, and temples actually suffer from migraine, muscle contraction headache, or one of the other chronic headache conditions. Even if your headaches happen to be associated with nasal symptoms, or occur most often during changes in weather, it is our opinion that so long as X rays do not show abnormalities of your sinuses, it is likely that your headaches are not sinus headaches.

If, however, diagnostic tests show that you do indeed have sinus disease, then you may require the care of a sinus specialist, known as an otorhinolaryngologist (oto-, ear; rhino-, nose; laryng-, throat; -ologist, specialist). You may need antibiotics for infection, in combination with potent decongestants and antihistamines. Occasionally, more complicated therapy requiring mechanical draining of the sinuses or even surgery becomes necessary.

Many patients have been told that their headaches are due to deviated septums and that surgical correction is recommended. It is our experience that only rarely has a deviated septum caused headaches or that headaches have been relieved by such surgery. Only when major abnormalities of the nasal structures are clearly demonstrated beforehand does surgery seem to help.

Finally, many people believe that their headaches are due to allergies. Unless you suffer from an obvious hay-fever-like reaction and your symptoms include sneezing, nasal discharge, and tearing, it is improbable that your headaches are due to allergy affecting your sinuses. If you do not suffer from these hay-fever-like symptoms, but your headaches seem to be related to eating certain foods or to an exposure to particular fumes or vapors, then it is possible that your symptoms are due not to an allergic response but to the effect that these substances have on your blood vessels (dilation).

Headaches following the drinking of alcohol or the eating of cheese or chocolate, for example, do not represent allergic reactions to these substances, but rather a physiological response to chemicals in these items. The difference in terminology may seem unimportant to you, but it has important biological implications. Nevertheless, in both situations the avoidance of the offending substances is worthwhile.

Chapter 6 Psychogenic Headaches: The Headaches for Which There Is No Apparent Physical Cause

In the late nineteenth century Sigmund Freud and others observed in some patients that when an emotional situation was resolved, a wide variety of physical symptoms, including headaches, seemed to disappear. From these important observations there has come an ever-increasing awareness of the power that the mind exerts over the body. The total extent of this influence is still not fully appreciated.

The emotional relationship to headaches is very important. We know that many of you have been told by your physicians that the cause of your headaches is emotional, suggesting that control over your emotions would diminish your headache problem. Many of you have greeted such an opinion with frustration or anger because the suggestion fails to acknowledge other important factors contributing to your discomfort. Just knowing that a headache is possible at any time in almost any situation can have a devastating impact upon your general feeling of tranquility. Indeed, many of you feel that a doctor's ascribing your headaches to emotional causes early in the interaction between you and the doctor represents an expedient, naive, and superficial interest in your problem.

Emotional factors do play an important role in triggering head-aches in many people. But even in these individuals, the actual role of emotion may be no more critical than several other important considerations, like hormonal, sleep-related, or nutritional factors. A quick diagnosis emphasizing emotions as the major trigger of headaches serves little therapeutic purpose and frequently inter-feres with the development of a good relationship between doctor and patient.

Emotional factors, like prolonged stress, anger, and internalized hostilities, can worsen many physical diseases, including headaches. In this sense, headaches represent psychosomatic illnesses.

The term psychosomatic (psycho-, mind; soma-, body) or psy-chophysiological (psycho-, mind; -physiological, body function) does not suggest that your symptoms are imaginary or "in your head." Instead, it suggests that an interaction between emotional and physical factors is evident. In psychosomatic or psychophysi-ological illnesses, emotional events significantly affect body physi-ology, and can occasionally cause very real and sometimes fatal physical illness. Among the psychosomatic or psychophysiological disorders are asthma, peptic ulcer, colitis (spasm, inflammation, and sometimes bleeding from the intestines), and perhaps some cases of hypertension (high blood pressure).

If you are skeptical about all of this, consider the significant effects that emotions have on your body when you are embar-rassed. If someone says a word that embarrasses you, it is not un-likely that you may experience a sudden blushing of your face, a physiological event caused by the sudden dilation of the blood vessels of the face, neck, and upper chest. If you are frightened, you will suddenly turn pale, your heart will beat rapidly, your brow may sweat, and your palms become clammy. These are physiological events that are *triggered* by emotional factors.

This concept is critical to our understanding of many cases of headaches. While it is true that many headaches have nothing to do with emotional events, and while some headaches are truly imaginary (see later in this chapter), many headaches are psycho-physiologically triggered. The headache is physical, but the trigger is emotional.

The reverse is also true. Emotional disturbances can result from having physical illnesses. When a patient suffers from persistent pain, each day can become an exercise in coping and avoiding activities or circumstances that trigger or amplify the discomfort. Reduced performance at work or in school can result from either the pain itself or the sedative effects of the medications used to control the pain. Absenteeism from work or school causes employers or teachers to lose patience, and complaining to family and friends may cause their eventual insensitivity, cynicism, and anger.

Fear that the unexplained and persistent pain comes from a serious disease compounds the problem. If the family doctor cannot help, the frustrating exercise of looking for a specialist or other medical help begins. Anxiety and desperation deepen. Doctors seeing your anxiety conclude that emotional upset is the *cause* of the headache problems, rather than the *result* of them. Eventually, in desperation, less conventional and sometimes unscientific methods of relief are tried. Bills accumulate. Side effects develop. Drug dependency may occur. Recurring pain can cause a deterioration in the quality of life, and the ensuing distress is an antecedent to even more pain. The pain causes more distress. And so the cycle continues.

What we are describing are two situations that can affect the headache sufferer. In the first, preexisting emotional disturbances trigger headaches that, like migraine, have physical explanations. If the headaches cannot be relieved, more emotional upset develops and more headaches are triggered.

In the second, physically explainable headaches that are not initially related to emotional circumstances eventually result in emotionally disruptive events and these trigger more headaches. In both circumstances, a disabling situation that is called the pain-distress cycle develops, and pain and distress interplay.

These two circumstances must be contrasted with a third situation. In this, there is no apparent physical basis for the headache. The pain exists, but there is no physical explanation, such as muscle contraction or vasodilation, to account for it. This type of headache is called the psychogenic (psycho-, mind; -genic, producing) headache, and its cause is based on complex mental processes. Another term for this condition is the nonorganic headache. Nonorganic, in this sense, means without physical (organic) changes. The psychogenic headache may represent a delusional or hallucinatory experience. The patient feels the pain, but there is no physical or biological explanation for it, at least based upon our current understanding.

An entirely satisfactory explanation for all cases of pain of non-organic origin does not exist at this time; however, the phenomenon called *somatization* appears relevant. Somatization is the process by which emotional sentiments are expressed or communicated with the "language" of body symptoms. In other words, the body learns to communicate for the mind.

Some examples may be helpful. A person with feelings of loneliness and depression may not be able to express these emotions verbally, but instead experiences pain and may communicate verbally "Oh, my head hurts so much I can't stand it." Anger at another individual may not be expressed as such but rather in the form of a disabling headache when an activity is planned with that individual. Young people may not be able to say that they do not want to go to school on a given day because of intimidation by friends, fear of failing tests, or because they are expected to stand up in front of the class and give a presentation. In fact, children may not even be in touch with why they do not want to go to school. Nevertheless, a child may wake up with a severe stomach ache, headache, or other symptoms and communicate to the mother how sick he or she feels. It is very important to emphasize that these examples do not necessarily represent conscious strategies, but rather have become, at least in many individuals, automatic, unconscious, and relatively uncontrollable experiences and methods of relating to other people.

Somatization is closely related to the mental mechanism of *conversion,* by which the mind converts emotional thoughts and conflicts into a variety of body symptoms, including pain. Numbness, loss of consciousness, and paralysis are but a few symptoms that in some individuals reflect conversion mechanisms. A full understanding of these complex mental functions is lacking, but a review of a few psychiatric principles will help clarify some of the issues.

It is believed that everyone harbors within his/her mind certain thoughts, inclinations, or temptations that tend to conflict with conscious moral beliefs. Some of these unconscious thoughts, many of which are of a sexual or aggressive nature, could be very upsetting if we were forced to recognize their existence within us. Ordinarily we are not troubled by these feelings because they are within the unconscious of our mind and we do not ordinarily feel conflict because we are not aware of these thoughts.

According to some psychiatric theories, these conflicts and feelings are effectively controlled by what are called mental defense mechanisms. These defense mechanisms work automatically to help maintain emotional stability by preventing us from coming into direct confrontation with our inner selves.

Some defense mechanisms are used daily and are considered normal. Others are rarely employed and only in very troubling circumstances. Conversion is one of the defense mechanisms that indicate the presence of more than the average strain and conflict. When an individual uses conversion, there is usually a very threatening emotional conflict at work. For reasons that are difficult to understand, the conflict is unconsciously *converted* into a symbolic, physical symptom.

Rationalization is a defense mechanism by which arguments are offered to ourselves and to others to justify, defend, or explain our behavior. The rationalization does not necessarily reflect the true reason for an action, but usually offers one that is acceptable. The defense mechanism is employed unconsciously, and when we rationalize, we almost always believe that the explanation or justification is valid.

Repression is another unconscious defense mechanism, and it is the act of "forgetting" events and circumstances that are emotionally painful. Many people block out emotionally painful experiences.

The following case history demonstrates the use of conversion, as well as two normal defense mechanisms, rationalization and repression.

A 22-year-old woman, who was raised in a deeply religious home that strongly disapproved of premarital sexual activity, fell in love with a man who, according to her, "persuaded" her to have sexual intercourse.

Though strong feelings of guilt were present, she rationalized the situation, insisting that she was in love and would someday marry this man. The woman further rationalized that society had become more tolerant about premarital sexual activity, and many of her girl friends were also involved in premarital sexual encounters. Her rationalizing helped her to accept her behavior and to keep her conflict discomfort under control.

Unfortunately, the close relationship with her lover eventually deteriorated and the couple separated. The woman was understandably upset, but she further rationalized that she was really better off, blaming the man for having coerced her into having sexual intercourse that she had not desired.

Within a week or two of the breakup, she claimed to have entirely "forgotten" (repressed) the love affair and the conflicts that it brought.

The woman tried to avoid becoming sexually involved with other men, but her sexual desires became overwhelming and she began to masturbate. First she masturbated only occasionally, but soon it was a frequent activity. She again rationalized that masturbation was "more decent" than sexual intercourse. Nevertheless, she became increasingly more disturbed by it because she continued to recall that her mother had once described masturbation as a "dirty, sinful, and immoral act," performed only by "sexual perverts."

One day, quite unexpectedly, the woman's right arm went limp and numb. As a result she stopped masturbating. For days she tried to ignore the paralysis and delayed seeing a physician. One of her friends commented that she seemed indifferent to what normally should have been a disturbing problem. Eventually, she did seek medical help.

The woman was examined by her family physician, who referred her to a neurologist. The neurologist found no physical basis for the paralysis and numbness in her right arm and made the diagnosis of a "conversion reaction." The patient was referred to a psychiatrist, and after months of therapy, her paralysis and numbness disappeared.

This young woman, without realizing it, used at least three important defense mechanisms. She used the "normal" defense mechanisms of rationalization and repression to help her handle the painful conflict of having sexual intercourse with a man who was not her husband. She used the "abnormal" defense mechanism of conversion to cope with her habit of masturbation: she converted the anguish caused by masturbating to a less emotionally painful experience—paralysis and numbness.

Conversion can also cause pain. The following case illustrates this.

A 35-year-old woman who considered oral sex to be immoral and sinful married a man who demanded oral sex. Although the woman protested, she nevertheless submitted to her husband's desires, "believing" that it was her duty and justifiable on that basis (rationalization).

Over a period of months, however, the woman began to experience increasingly severe and frequent headaches. At first her headaches did not interfere with sexual activity, but eventually they became so intense and constant that all sexual interaction ceased.

She did not seek medical help immediately, often "joking" to her husband that she probably had a brain tumor. (This concern is common to many patients with frequent headaches, but in this patient, guilt and punishment fantasies might have motivated some of her feelings.) Finally, the woman sought medical help.

Many tests were performed, and finally the woman was told that no physical basis for her headaches could be found. The woman was referred to a psychiatrist who focused on the conflict between her submissive sexual conduct and her strong feelings of guilt and revulsion about oral sex. After months of therapy, the headaches vanished and she resumed having a mutually satisfactory sexual relationship with her husband.

A variety of emotional circumstances in addition to the conflicts and guilt suggested by the above examples may be important in conversion and somatization. These include depression, anger, anxiety, internalized hostility, and rage.

Although the nonorganic headache has no apparent physical basis, the headache is nonetheless very painful. But unlike most cases of migraine or muscle contraction headaches, these headaches do not demonstrate reliably present features or patterns except that the pain is often constant and usually unresponsive to all medications.

Keep in mind that some patients with muscle contraction headaches and migraine also suffer prolonged and continued attacks, and some of these headaches may not completely respond to medications either. Your doctor must distinguish between these very difficult migraine and muscle contraction cases and those of a nonorganic basis.

The nonorganic headache is not easily diagnosed. A firm diagnosis cannot be established until the physician has considered the more likely possibility that the pain is due to a less typical or unresponsive form of migraine or muscle contraction headache. Even though from your medical history a physician might suspect a nonorganic headache early in the course of the work-up, it is likely that a variety of analgesics, tranquilizing drugs, antidepressants, and sometimes antimigraine medications will be tried in an effort to relieve the pain. When emotional factors are responsible, efforts to relieve the discomfort with medications invariably fail.

Abuse of medication is a major problem encountered in persons suffering from psychogenic headaches. And very often, all analgesic medications must be discontinued before relief can be achieved. Dr. Lee Kudrow of California believes that *only* if analgesics are completely avoided is there any real chance of relieving the conversion headache.

In support of the premise that medications may cause or add to emotional problems is the fact that certain drugs may cause or worsen depression. Examples of these are certain blood-pressure-reducing drugs, antianxiety drugs (tranquilizers), and even birth-control pills in some women. Additional biological causes of depression include viral infections, certain glandular abnormalities, nutritional deficiency, and even some anemias (reduced blood count).

Finally, let us summarize what we are trying to emphasize in this chapter. Emotion plays an important role in the triggering of physiological events, some of which can cause significant illnesses, among them chronic pain. We call these headaches psychophysiological or psychosomatic, because the mind triggers the physiology that causes the pain. Numerous other biological factors may well play a role in the predisposition toward these illnesses, but the mind and its distress can aggravate the process.

This situation is to be contrasted with those headaches that are truly rooted in emotional illness. In such cases, the headache is hallucinatory or delusional; the patient imagines the presence of pain. The patient experiences discomfort, but the discomfort represents a poorly understood phenomenon in which pain occurs without apparent physiological change. Someday we will understand this better, perhaps when we understand more about the endorphins and the other chemical agents of the brain that may be altered in the presence of emotional distress. For the time being, however, these headaches are considered different from those that we currently call migraine, muscle contraction, and the other chronic headache disorders.

An accurate diagnosis and successful therapy for nonorganic headaches usually require both neurological and psychiatric assistance. After the diagnosis is clearly established, the therapy must confront the emotions responsible for the headaches. Only then can the appropriate methods of treatment be undertaken, and only then will there be a chance that the headaches will subside and eventually vanish.

At the end of this chapter you will find a quiz to informally test yourself for depression. You may wish to take this quiz. Please remember, however, that simply being depressed and also having headaches does not mean that your headaches are nonorganic. Both migraine and muscle contraction headaches seem to worsen when depression is present.

A DEPRESSION QUIZ

This quiz is designed to assist you, in an informal way, to determine if elements of depression are within you. Most people possess at least some of these elements, even when they are not depressed.

After finishing the quiz, compare your answers to those in the Answer Key. The answers listed in the key represent the choices that indicate a depressive response. The more your answers match the indicated responses, the more likely it is that your behavior is influenced by depression.

Answer the following questions Yes or No.

	Yes	No
1. Are you looking forward to future events?	——	——
2. Do you have plans for your next vacation?	——	——
3. Do you believe that next year will bring better tidings for you than this year?	——	——
4. Have you lost interest in hobbies and events that once occupied you?	——	——
5. Do you have confidence in yourself?	——	——
6. Are you angry with or disappointed in yourself even if you do not know why?	——	——
7. Do you have significant unexplained mood swings, being happy and elated at one moment and then sad tearful and lonely the next?	——	——
8. Do you feel a sense of impending doom?	——	——
9. Do you awake early in the morning (4:00 or 5:00 A.M.) for no apparent reason and are unable to go back to sleep?	——	——
10. Have you lost your appetite?	——	——
11. Have you lost weight recently?	——	——
12. Do you laugh heartily at anything anymore?	——	——
13. Do you find it almost impossible to concentrate?	——	——
14. Do you burst into tears for no special reason?	——	——
15. Have you lost your incentive to perform your tasks and responsibilities?	——	——
16. Have you noticed that you are taking greater risks and less concerned about your welfare?	——	——
17. Do you sit and wring your hands?	——	——
18. Are you troubled by many uncomfortable thoughts coming to mind?	——	——
19. Have you reached the conclusion that you just cannot cope?	——	——
20. Has anyone in your family been hospitalized for depression or mania?	——	——
21. Do you prefer to be alone?	——	——
22. Have you lost your interest in sex?	——	——
23. Does life seem worth living?	——	——

	Yes	No
24. Have you considered suicide as a means of escaping?	——	——
25. Have you lost interest in friends recently?	——	——

Compare your answers to those in the following Answer Key. We must remind you that a simple quiz of this type cannot be considered an accurate assessment of your mood. However, the more your answers coincide with the depressive responses in the key, the more likely it is that you are experiencing some degree of depression. If your answers do reflect a depressed state, particularly if you have answered Questions 23 and 24 with depressive responses, we urge you to seek medical help immediately. Chances are excellent that with the assistance of a qualified professional, the cloud under which you live can be lifted and a new and exciting chapter in your life may begin. Your headaches may vanish as well.

There is a difference between grieving following a great and important loss, such as the death of someone you love, and the illness called depression. Grieving over a real loss is not only expected but is important in resolving the loss of someone or something important to you. Depression, on the other hand, may occur without any apparent provocation, and its duration and intensity can be much longer and more profound than grieving. If your answers to the quiz indicate a depressive trend, but if you have recently suffered a great loss, you may be experiencing a grief response rather than depression. In either case, however, you may be helped if you seek qualified professional assistance.

Answer Key

The following answers are the depressive responses. The more of your answers that coincide with these, the more likely is the chance that you are depressed.

1. No.
2. No.

3. No.
4. Yes.
5. No.
6. Yes.
7. Yes.
8. Yes.
9. Yes.
10. Yes.
11. Yes.
12. No.
13. Yes.
14. Yes.
15. Yes.
16. Yes.
17. Yes.
18. Yes.
19. Yes.
20. Yes.
21. Yes.
22. Yes.
23. No.
24. Yes.
25. Yes.

Chapter 7 Headaches as Symptoms of Other Medical Conditions

In this chapter we will discuss a group of headaches that are referred to as the secondary headache conditions. These headaches develop as the result of, or secondary to, one or more of a wide variety of medical problems that range from mild and benign conditions to very severe and sometimes life-threatening illnesses. Ironically, many serious medical problems cause head pain that is very mild when compared to the discomfort of a bad migraine or a cluster headache. And many very benign medical conditions are capable of causing very severe head pain.

When you seek medical attention for your headaches, your physician must determine whether or not your headaches reflect the presence of a serious disease. This task is not always easy, which is why it is often necessary to perform numerous tests.

This chapter does not discuss all the illnesses that can cause headaches, because almost any of the known medical disorders can provoke head pain. We have chosen a group of headaches and the illnesses that cause them that occur very frequently, are terribly misunderstood, or are of particular interest.

INFECTION

Few of us have escaped the nagging headache that can accompany a cold or other infection. Headache is only one of the uncomfortable symptoms associated with infections, but head pain may be so severe that medical attention for the headache itself becomes necessary.

The exact mechanism by which an infection throughout the body and the accompanying fever cause headache is not fully understood. It is likely that the head pain is due to either or both the inflammation of sensitive structures or the dilation of the blood vessels that invariably occurs when the body temperature goes up.

Blood vessel dilation develops automatically during fever and is nature's way of cooling the body by transferring some blood from internal regions to the skin, where it is exposed to air and thus cooled. The headache due to fever may resemble migraine because both are related to blood vessel dilation. The pain is often pounding, frequently hurts behind the eyes, and is aggravated by a sudden change in position, particularly bending over.

A headache that comes as part of a generalized infection and fever may be successfully treated by reducing the fever with medications like aspirin and acetaminophen or by resorting to a variety of home remedies such as cool baths or alcohol rubs. Aspirin and acetaminophen, of course, have both pain-relieving and temperature-lowering properties. Aspirin is best in this situation, however, because it has an ability to reduce inflammation which acetaminophen lacks.

MENINGITIS

Headaches regularly accompany meningitis. Meningitis means an inflammation of the meninges, the tissue covering the brain. This inflammation usually results from infection, but other causes exist as well. This section will discuss meningitis caused by infection.

When meningitis is caused by a simple virus, the condition is not usually serious. Viral meningitis is often part of a generalized viral infection, like a cold, although most colds do not cause significant involvement of the brain or its covering. Exactly why some viral infections cause meningitis is not known.

Viral meningitis usually brings with it a severe headache and an uncomfortable sensitivity to light called photophobia. Most patients also experience a very stiff neck. The stiff neck occurs because the meninges that surround the spinal cord in the neck region are inflamed.

A headache brought on by viral meningitis usually lasts only a few days, but it can be very painful and relief may require very strong analgesics. The viral infection responsible for the meningitis does not usually require antibiotics and in most cases will improve in a week or so.

Viral infections cannot usually be treated with antibiotics. Antibiotics are used when bacteria, like streptococcus (a "strep" infection) or staphylococcus (a "staph" infection) are the cause of the illness. For the most part, the body's own defenses are able to fight off viral infections.

Meningitis produced by a bacterial infection also causes headache and stiff neck, but unlike its viral counterpart, bacterial meningitis is a serious and life-threatening condition that requires prompt antibiotic therapy. Bacterial meningitis, often referred to as "spinal meningitis," is associated with many serious neurological problems. At the time the stiff neck and headache first appear, however, the victim may not seem particularly ill, but hours later coma may occur.

Stiff neck and headache do not always indicate the presence of meningitis. A strained neck, cervical arthritis, or the overall achiness and stiffness accompanying colds that do not invade the nervous system may also produce headache and stiffness of the neck. Sometimes, tumors in the neck or the back of the brain can cause similar symptoms. A prompt medical evaluation of all cases of stiff neck is obviously very important.

BRAIN TUMOR

Headaches can accompany some brain tumors, and people suffering from recurring or severe headaches are often quite concerned that they have a tumor. But it is rare for headaches that recur for several years to be due to a tumor, no matter how severe the head pain is. Headaches usually do not occur until late in the course of most brain tumors, after many other symptoms have developed. Some patients with brain tumors do not experience headache at all.

The headache of a brain tumor does not have any particular characteristic to identify it. The pain may be over the entire head or localized in a special area. It is frequently a dull pain and may be very mild, and it may last for only moments at a time or be continuous.

The headache due to a brain tumor rarely awakens people during sleep, as migraine or cluster headaches do. Movement of the head and changes in posture may increase the discomfort, but this characteristic is shared by many other headaches, like migraine and the headache associated with fever. The brain tumor headache may be eased temporarily by simple analgesics, such as aspirin. For this reason alone, the prolonged use of analgesics for undiagnosed headache is clearly unwise.

Pseudotumor Cerebri—Pseudotumor cerebri literally defined means a false tumor of the brain. Although less than an ideal name for a medical problem, the disorder represents a condition in which there occurs an increase of pressure inside the skull. What distinguishes this condition from many other disorders that cause an increase of pressure, such as a brain tumor, is the absence of any identifiable abnormality of the brain tissue. A person affected with pseudotumor cerebri, more recently called "benign intracranial hypertension," will experience headache as the major symptom of the condition. If the disorder is allowed to worsen for a prolonged period of time, a reduction of vision and ultimate blindness can occur.

The headache associated with pseudotumor cerebri is usually of a nonspecific nature. It is constant and not terribly intense. Pain in the forehead region, behind the eyes, and over the top of the head is common. Interestingly, most but not all persons affected by this disorder are overweight women.

The cause of pseudotumor cerebri remains obscure. In some cases, it has been associated with the use of birth-control pills and other hormone substances (such as cortisone), the taking of a urinary antibiotic called naladixic acid, being pregnant, being obese, or having anemia or low calcium in the blood. Other glandular problems have also been associated with the disorder. In children, pseudotumor cerebri has been observed when tetracycline or too much or too little vitamin A is ingested.

Most cases of pseudotumor cerebri occur without identifiable cause and, as mentioned, the patients are often overweight women. The diagnosis is established by observing swelling of the optic nerves by looking into the eyes with an ophthalmoscope. The increase in pressure is confirmed by performing a lumbar puncture, after tests to rule out a brain tumor and other various conditions have been performed. If the diagnosis is made early in the course of the illness and before visual damage occurs, pseudotumor cerebri can be easily treated by reducing the pressure inside the skull with the use of special medications. In most instances, pseudotumor cerebri does not pose any serious threat to life or health, unless, of course, it is allowed to worsen over months and years.

STROKE (CEREBROVASCULAR ACCIDENT)

Although "stroke" is not a precise medical term, the word refers to sudden neurological impairment due to a blocked blood vessel in a particular area of the brain. The most common symptoms of stroke are weakness and loss of sensation on one side of the body. The symptoms of a stroke are caused by the loss of function of a particular portion of the brain, the portion not receiving adequate blood due to the blockage.

Headache is sometimes the sign of an impending stroke. Headache may also follow a stroke. But these headaches have no special characteristics, so they are rarely of help in warning of or diagnosing the stroke.

Occasionally a blood vessel within the substance of the brain or near its surface can rupture. This usually causes a sudden and severe headache. The headache is often followed by loss of consciousness, along with other neurological symptoms.

If blood from a ruptured blood vessel seeps into the space around the brain and travels between the meninges down to the neck area, it may cause irritation of the meninges with an accompanying stiff neck. Bleeding into or around the brain is a life-threatening condition, and it may require immediate surgical intervention.

Headaches beginning in late life may warn that the brain is not getting enough oxygen. This can occur as a result of lung disease, heart disease, hardening of the arteries (atherosclerosis or arteriosclerosis), or a number of other conditions that deprive the brain of oxygen. The pain from this oxygen deficiency does not have any special characteristics. The cause may be blood vessel widening (dilation) in an attempt to bring more blood to the oxygen-starved tissue.

HYPERTENSION (HIGH BLOOD PRESSURE)

Hypertension means elevated blood pressure; it does not mean increased emotional tension. Many patients wrongly believe that the stress or anxiety associated with a visit to a doctor's office can raise normal blood pressure to *significantly* high levels. This is not usually the case.

Although very high blood pressure does cause headache, head pain rarely results from small to moderately elevated blood pressure. There is, however, a higher than average incidence of hypertension in patients who also experience migraine.

The headache associated with significant hypertension is often felt in the back of the head and neck, and can be worsened by movement. It may be most severe upon awakening in the morning. (Morning headaches also occur in migraine and muscle contraction headache conditions.)

When hypertension causes the headache, treating the elevated blood pressure often will relieve the discomfort. But some of the drugs used in the treatment of hypertension can act in a way to cause headaches.

Hypertension is a potentially serious problem. If high blood pressure is present for a long time (a few years), it will injure the heart, blood vessels, and kidneys, and predispose the victim to stroke and heart attack. Lowering of blood pressure before this damage occurs is an important aspect of preventive medicine.

HEAD INJURY OR HEAD TRAUMA

In addition to the immediate pain following an injury involving the head, a more prolonged and enduring headache may develop. This headache can start at the time of injury or several hours or days later. This persistent headache can be either mild or severe.

Why a prolonged headache follows head injury is not entirely known, but damage to the scalp and its muscles, the nerves and blood vessels, the meninges, and the spine and its muscles may all play a role. Injury to the blood vessels of the scalp and meninges can cause a loss of their ability to dilate and constrict appropriately, resulting in a headache that is similar in some ways to migraine and other vascular headaches. This headche may be pounding and may become worse with exertion or changes in posture. The pounding will sometimes awaken its victim at night. This headache may respond to simple analgesics or may require stronger medication or antimigraine medications.

The force of a blow to the head is very often transmitted to the neck, causing injury to the vertebrae, nerves, spinal cord, and muscles and tendons. The injury may trigger the neck muscles to contract painfully. This posttraumatic headache is similar in many ways to other muscle contraction or vascular headaches. It may be treated by relaxing the muscle spasm and controlling the excessive blood vessel dilation. Biofeedback, protective collars, and medications used for migraine and muscle contraction headaches are frequently effective. If there is a possibility of injury to vertebrae, nerves, or spinal cord, consultation with a neurologist or neurosurgeon may be necessary.

When nerves are injured, pain and tingling may be transmitted to the shoulders, arms, and hands. Weakness and strange sensations like numbness and tingling can also occur if there is compression of nerve tissues. The pain of an injured neck may be referred to the top or the back of the head because the neck nerves also supply these areas. (See Appendix.)

Injury to the scalp and the scars that ultimately form can lead to pain that seems to arise from inside the skull but which actually comes from the injured scalp itself. Successful treatment of this discomfort can sometimes be achieved by "freezing" the injured tissue with a local anesthetic or alcohol. If this fails to bring relief, cutting a nerve to a small area of the scalp may be helpful.

A condition called the "posttraumatic syndrome" deserves special mention. This disorder may occur after an accident or criminal assault. The condition can follow even a mild injury of the head and includes a variety of symptoms: headaches, dizziness, irritability, insomnia, anxiety, depression, and reduced ability to concentrate. Sometimes, a personality change occurs as well. These symptoms may last weeks, months, or even years, but significant abnormalities are not usually found to account for them. Nevertheless, the fear that brain injury has occurred frequently adds to the emotional distress already present with this condition.

The treatment of posttraumatic syndrome includes reassurance that no serious damage has occurred, sedation, and often antidepressant medication. Sometimes there is no response to treatment and the symptoms continue until they finally disappear months or years later.

The severity of the trauma does not seem to be the factor that determines the intensity of the symptoms in the posttraumatic syndrome. The personality of the victim before the head injury is very important in determining the intensity of the symptoms and the emotional response to the injury. If a person is tense, anxious, or depressed, it is likely that these symptoms will be heightened.

Studies over the years suggest that when financial compensation for injury or when legal matters concerning the trauma are pending, the symptoms following even mild head injury may be of longer duration and of greater intensity. Self-employed people, with little to gain from weeks or months of disability, and athletes, who often suffer many body and head injuries, appear to be less prone to many of the unpleasant symptoms seen in other groups of people who have suffered minor head injury. Cynical as this statement may seem to you, medical evidence strongly supports these conclusions.

All cases of head injury deserve prompt medical evaluation. Even mild blows to the head can result in blood clots, seizures, coma, and even death.

TOXINS AND MEDICATIONS

It is practically impossible to avoid exposure to the myriad of toxins and noxious vapors present in our technological society. We encounter them daily in industry, agriculture, and the home. Many of these agents either have been proved harmful or are strongly suspected of causing many illnesses, including headache.

One group of chemicals particularly likely to produce headache is the organic solvents. Included in this group are turpentine, carbon tetrachloride, benzine (used in gasoline), and benzene (used in leather processing, motor fuels, dyes, glue, paints, and linoleums). Mild exposure to these substances may bring on only a headache, but long or daily exposure can cause serious medical problems.

Formaldehyde is another substance that can cause headaches as well as other symptoms if exposure is prolonged. Headaches have been reported in people whose homes were recently insulated with insulation containing formaldehyde.

The metal lead—not graphite, as in "lead" pencils—can cause serious neurological impairment. Lead is particularly harmful to children. Excessive ingestion causes convulsions, brain swelling, and coma. A major reason for lead intoxication in children is ingestion of lead-containing paint chips from walls or toys. In adults as well as children, lead ingestion can come from contact with the chemicals in lead batteries, dabbing an art brush dipped in lead-containing paint on the tongue, or drinking moonshine whiskey when lead pipes or lead solder was used in the tubing system. Drinking from glazed pottery not properly baked or living near air- and water-polluting industries may also cause excessive exposure to lead. Children and adults with unexplained headaches should have a test for lead intoxication.

Carbon monoxide gas is a poisonous, odorless substance, and it can be a source of headaches. Thus, if headaches develop in auto mechanics, roadside toll booth operators, people who drive on expressways for long hours, or anyone who might be exposed to carbon monoxide fumes, this cause of headaches should be considered. Similarly, during the winter months, when furnaces are on, unexplained headaches may be caused by faulty furnaces emitting carbon monoxide gas.

Headaches caused by carbon monoxide usually improve when exposure to the gas is altered. In cases of mild intoxication, permanent injury does not occur, but brain damage as well as death can result from prolonged or intense exposure.

Many medications, including some used to treat headaches, can themselves cause the head to ache. Among these medications are various drugs used to treat epilepsy and a variety of drugs used to treat hypertension, including any that contain the blood-pressure-lowering agents reserpine, hydralazine, or certain diuretics. The antidepressants, particularly the monoamine oxidase inhibitors mentioned in Chapter 3, may also cause headaches in some people, but they are used to treat headache conditions in others.

Indomethacin (Indocin), a drug used to treat arthritis, may be quite effective in controlling certain types of headaches, even though one of its side effects is headache. Nitroglycerin and other nitrite-containing substances as well as medications that dilate blood vessels are capable of triggering headaches. Dilating medications are used to treat heart pain (angina pectoris) and other circulatory problems due to arteriosclerosis (atherosclerosis [hardening of the arteries]). Amphetamines, as well as other stimulants, ephedrine (a decongestant), some asthma drugs, and diet pills can and do produce headaches in some people.

Caffeine is added to many over-the-counter and prescription medications. Caffeine acts as a stimulant and affects the blood vessels, constricting some and dilating others. In small doses, caffeine can be helpful in relieving some headaches, although its proven efficacy remains in doubt. But when too much caffeine is consumed, preexisting headaches can be worsened. Too much caffeine can cause headaches even where there was no headache before. Overconsumption of caffeine can easily result from taking caffeine-containing medication, such as Fiorinal, Cafergot, Darvon Compound, Norgesic, Excedrin, Anacin, Vanquish, and others, together with the daily intake of foods and beverages that contain caffeine, such as coffee, tea, cola, and chocolate.

In addition to causing or intensifying headaches, caffeine can produce headaches if withdrawal from it occurs after an individual has become dependent on it. We believe that when there is a background of consuming an overabundance of caffeine during the day, some morning headaches are withdrawal headaches, created by withdrawal of caffeine during the eight or more hours of sleep. If you abuse caffeine (the term "abuse" is appropriate because caffeine is a drug) and if you have headaches, you might get substantial relief by gradually reducing your total caffeine consumption. A more complete discussion of caffeine and its effects can be found in Chapter 9.

TEMPORAL ARTERITIS

There are two temporal arteries, one on each side of the forehead in the temple area. The temporal arteries can be felt by pressing your fingers against your temples and feeling for pulsations. Arteritis means inflammation of an artery, and when inflammation occurs, the blood vessel swells. When there is a severe swelling, the blood flow through the artery is blocked.

Temporal arteritis is not fully understood, but in this disorder the temporal arteries, as well as many other arteries in the head, become obstructed by inflammation. The blocked arteries impede or stop blood flow to the brain. Temporal arteritis is a serious disorder that usually affects people over the age of fifty, although there are younger victims. Headache can be one of the early symptoms of temporal arteritis, but blindness and stroke may follow if the condition is not treated promptly. Occasionally joint and muscle pain throughout the entire body also occurs.

Temporal arteritis should be considered as a possible diagnosis for anyone over fifty years of age who suffers from unexplained headaches. The inflammation can be reduced by cortisone-like drugs. When the inflammation subsides and blood flow is restored, the headache pain will recede and the possibility of blindness and stroke will be reduced.

DISEASE OF THE EYES

Pain from disease in or around the eyes may be referred to other regions of the head or face. Conversely, pain from another area of the head may be felt in the eye area. People seeking relief for headaches often first explore the need for glasses or a change in lenses before seeking a more thorough medical evaluation.

Before discussing diseases of the eyes and the headaches that they can cause, the roles of ophthalmologist, optometrist, and optician should be clarified, since people seeking help for problems with their sight or eyes may not understand the differences among these specialties. An ophthalmologist is a physician who has graduated from medical school and has specialized in diseases of the eyes and related structures. An ophthalmologist diagnoses and treats conditions of the eyes, and, when necessary, performs surgery. He/she also evaluates the need for lenses. An optometrist is not a doctor of medicine and is primarily concerned with evaluating and measuring the need for glasses. The optometrist makes lenses and dispenses them. The optometrist can also examine the eyes for certain diseases and then refer the patient to an ophthalmologist for treatment. An optician fills prescriptions for lenses and dispenses and repairs frames. All three professionals play an important and complementary role in the care of the eyes.

We believe that the vast majority of people with chronic head pain around the forehead or eye area have migraine or muscle contraction headaches. But, because a disease of the eyes may be to blame, it is appropriate that a thorough examination of the eye structures be carried out. Although optometrists are well trained for what they do, a thorough evaluation for certain diseases of the eyes is best performed by an ophthalmologist, whose training also includes disorders of the brain, some of which can cause headaches.

Eyestrain can cause headaches. This is particularly common following long periods of reading in poor light. Eyestrain is most common when there is a subtle or more noticeable weakness and imbalance of the eye movement muscles or ability to focus. Glaring and bright light may also produce discomfort. Fluorescent lighting may create an unnoticed flickering in lighting intensity, and headaches can be the result of this.

The pain of eyestrain is usually located around the eyes and forehead, frequently improving after reading is discontinued and the eyes are rested. Improving lighting conditions or obtaining eyeglasses or a new prescription will often be of some relief.

While poor focusing ability can cause headaches, many more people believe that they need glasses in order to stop their headaches than is actually the case. Many patients report that when the glasses are acquired and used, no improvement in the headaches is noticed.

We believe that it is unlikely that your headaches will benefit from wearing glasses if you have headaches at times other than just when reading and if you do not experience focusing problems. To prevent the needless purchase of expensive eyeglasses, we suggest that you get two independent opinions and ask each doctor to give you the recommended lens prescription after the examination. Compare from one doctor to the next. (An excellent discussion of this subject can be found in *Consumer Reports*, November 1977.)

Glaucoma is a serious disease of the eyes that is capable of causing headaches as well as blindness. Sometimes the disease remains silent until damage is done. Glaucoma may strike the young as well as the old. The symptoms associated with glaucoma are due to impaired drainage of fluid from the eyes. The reduced drainage causes pressure within the eyes, and it is this increased pressure that leads to damage if the condition is not corrected.

Pain from glaucoma may be severe or mild. It is felt in or around one or both eyes or forehead, and nausea and vomiting may be present. Many individuals suffering from glaucoma see colored halos around lighted objects or experience a mistiness of vision.

A test for glaucoma can be performed simply and painlessly in a doctor's office by using a device that measures the pressure within the eyes. All adults should have a yearly test for the disease.

Depending upon the severity and type of glaucoma, the condition can be treated with medication or by surgery.

Individuals with certain types of glaucoma must avoid those drugs known to worsen the disorder. Among these are antihistamines, some bowel relaxants, the tricyclic antidepressants, some anti-nauseants, certain tranquilizers, and some drugs used in Parkinson's disease. Over-the-counter pain or headache preparations may contain these or similar agents and should be avoided until you consult your doctor. It is particularly important for you to have your eyes checked for glaucoma if you must take one of these drugs for prolonged periods.

Tumors and infections of the eyes may also cause headaches. These and other diseases of the eyes, however, are infrequent causes of recurring head pain. Again, it should be emphasized that anyone experiencing headache of uncertain cause should be evaluated for glaucoma as well as for other serious illnesses of the eyes.

DENTAL PROBLEMS AND EAR DISEASE

Pain arising from the mouth, ear, or jaw can be referred to another part of the head and be felt as headache pain. Infections of the gum, arthritis of the jaw, or a poor dental alignment may cause head pain. Some people who have sought medical doctors' help for headaches find that the cause of the pain is of dental origin, but many more people who have actually suffered from migraine or cluster headaches have made vain attempts to find relief by undergoing tooth extractions.

The temporomandibular joint, or jaw joint, is located just in front of the ear canal. You can feel it moving by placing a finger immediately in front of an ear while opening and closing your mouth. Arthritis of this joint, jaw clenching, teeth gnashing, or misalignment and imbalance of bite can all be responsible for causing headache. This pain may be due to inflammation or stress in the jaw joint or on the jaw muscles. It may radiate down the neck into a shoulder, in or behind an ear, or upward into the temple region. Feeling or hearing a cracking noise when chewing may indicate that you have an abnormality of the temporomandibular joint.

Some patjents who suffer from headaches due to jaw abnormalities have found relief by placing specially designed and fitted mouthpiece devices between their teeth at night, or by undergoing certain special procedures performed by professionals skilled in treating diseases of the temporomandibular joint.

Currently, it is claimed by some that temporomandibular (TM) joint dysfunction is responsible for most chronic headaches and atypical facial pain. Such a claim, in our opinion, represents a gross overstatement that at this time is unsupported by objective data. Although it is true that some patients with chronic head pain experience their pain as a result of malocclusion or some other abnormality of the mouth, teeth, or jaw, we believe that most people who have minor alterations of their TM joint or bite do not experience pain as a consequence. (Rarely, pain in the TM joint may be associated with rheumatoid arthritis, but there is usually involvement of other joints of the body as well.) We recommend delaying the often expensive treatment programs to correct the bite until confirmatory opinions have been obtained and more traditional and accepted diagnoses have been ruled out.

HYPOGLYCEMIA

Hypoglycemia means abnormally low blood sugar. Over the past few years there has been increased public concern about this disease. Some of this publicity has been generated by unscientific literature proposing that a wide variety of otherwise unexplained symptoms is actually caused by low blood sugar.

While it is quite true that hypoglycemia can cause many and varied symptoms, the frequency of hypoglycemia's actually causing all of the complaints ascribed to it is minimal. Simply feeling hungry does not necessarily mean that your blood sugar is abnormally low. Healthy patients deprived of food for many days do not become hypoglycemic, because a normal liver will store the products necessary to form sugar (glucose) and maintain a reasonably normal level of blood sugar for long periods of time without food.

An individual does not have to be hypoglycemic in order to experience a headache when meals are missed or when he/she is hungry. You may recall that in Chapter 2, on migraine, we mentioned that going five hours or longer between meals could provoke a migraine attack in people not hypoglycemic. A nonmigraine headache may also develop when meals are missed.

When true hypoglycemia does occur, symptoms may include not only headache but light-headedness, dizziness, trembling, and sweating. When severe, loss of consciousness, convulsions, and even death may ensue.

Individuals experiencing headache or other unexplained symptoms when there are long gaps between meals should nevertheless be evaluated for hypoglycemia. Hypoglycemia may be an early symptom of diabetes mellitus, a disease in which the pancreas cannot produce necessary amounts of insulin, so that very high blood sugar levels occur. The headaches that result from long gaps between meals can often be avoided by eating four to six well-spaced meals per day and avoiding certain foods that promote a dramatic elevation and then a rapid fall of the blood sugar level. Foods that are inclined to do this usually contain large amounts of sugar (carbohydrate, starch). It is far better to eat small amounts of food frequently than to overload your system by eating one or two large meals a day.

If you have headaches upon awaking in the morning, you might try eating a protein snack at bedtime. Although many headaches not related to sugar levels occur in the morning, if you customarily do not eat between dinner the night before and breakfast the next day, a fast of possibly twelve hours, eating at bedtime a small protein snack that will digest slowly may help avoid morning headaches. Eating any food high in sugar or starch at bedtime is not appropriate since this is likely to produce a rapid rise and then a fall in the sugar level while you sleep, making your body even more vulnerable to headache by early morning.

We must emphasize, once again, that simply because eating a low-carbohydrate snack prior to bedtime helps to prevent the nighttime or morning attack of pain, it does not necessarily indicate the presence of hypoglycemia.

The symptoms of hypoglycemia can be very similar to the symptoms of anxiety. These may include, as mentioned earlier, sweating, lightheadedness, dizziness, trembling, and even fainting.

A recent study showed that most patients who thought they were experiencing hypoglycemia were actually experiencing anxiety attacks. This important observation is quite consistent with the belief of most physicians who feel that the incidence of hypoglycemia has been significantly exaggerated in the minds of the public.

LUMBAR PUNCTURE (SPINAL TAP) HEADACHE

Like so many other topics concerning headaches, considerable misunderstanding surrounds the subject of spinal taps. The method by which a spinal tap is performed is explained in Chapter 8. The procedure itself does not cause the headache, but the effects of removing the fluid can.

The tissue that produces the spinal fluid is capable of replenishing the total volume of fluid at least three times a day. Nevertheless, when spinal fluid is removed, a temporary reduction of volume does exit. Additionally, a small and minor leakage of fluid may occur through the hole made by the needle for a short time after the test. Although this is not a medically serious problem, a headache can be produced by the resulting lowered fluid pressure. A headache caused by the drop in spinal fluid pressure is made worse when the patient is standing or sitting and can be relieved or improved by reclining.

The spinal tap headache does not usually appear until hours after the procedure has been completed. It lasts for about two or three days, or occasionally longer. Although uncomfortable, the condition is not serious.

It is advisable to recline for a few hours immediately after the spinal tap. This can help prevent or relieve the headache.

A spinal tap is not always followed by a headache, but because of an almost universal concern that a headache will occur, the anticipation that a headache will develop may play a role in causing one. During my (J.R.S.) internship, a spinal tap was to be performed on a very suggestible patient. Upon feeling the needle enter her skin and before the removal of even one drop of fluid, the patient screamed, "I'm getting my headache already." Although the patient was reassured that the spinal tap could not yet have been responsible for her headache discomfort, the patient persisted and the spinal tap was canceled.

THE EXERTIONAL HEADACHE

During the past year, Dr. Seymour Diamond and his associate Dr. Jose Medina, both noted headache authorities in Chicago, have identified the presence of an "exertional" headache that tends to occur in some individuals following or during periods of extreme exertion. This headache entity has formerly been known under various other titles, including the *cough headache, sneeze headache, lifting headache, stooping headache, laughter headache, yawn headache,* and so on. The headache itself tends to have a throbbing, sharp, or stabbing quality. It may last minutes to hours and usually occurs in patients with preexisting headaches. It is occasionally accompanied by other symptoms.

It is very important, however, when patients experience head pain during periods of exertion, that a careful assessment be made to rule out significant neurological illnesses that can cause such pain. While the exertional headache is probably very common in patients who are otherwise healthy, serious and life-threatening illnesses may also produce this symptom and should not be overlooked.

The treatment for the exertional headache can include avoidance of the aggravating activity and the use of antimigraine medication. Drs. Diamond and Medina suggest the use of indomethacin (Indocin), the antiarthritic medicine useful in some other headache disorders.

TRIGEMINAL NEURALGIA (TIC DOULOUREUX)

The trigeminal nerve, which is the fifth cranial nerve (see Appendix), carries sensation for much of the head and nearly all of the face. It also is the nerve that carries impulses to the muscles of chewing and jaw movement. Neuralgia means pain of a major nerve, although the term is often incorrectly used to describe vague aches and pains throughout the body.

Trigeminal neuralgia is a painful condition that usually develops after the age of forty, but which can occur earlier. The pain involves a portion of one side of the face and is lightninglike and stabbing. The cheek, chin, gum, or forehead may be involved. Each bout of the recurring, repetitive pain usually lasts only minutes but can be excruciating.

Characteristic of this condition is that the painful episodes can be activated by a trigger point located somewhere on the face or in the mouth. This trigger area is often so sensitive that even the lightest touch or a puff of wind starts the attack. Many persons avoid chewing food or brushing their teeth on the involved side of the mouth; others will not wash their face, and men who are affected will not shave on the sensitive side.

The reason for this condition is still unknown. A virus infection of the nerve, compression of the nerve by pulsating blood vessels, and other theories have been suggested. Successful treatment is usually available; either medication or surgery can bring relief to most people with this condition. Trigeminal neuralgia usually abates spontaneously in a few weeks or months after the attack begins, but persistent attacks can occur and a recurrence of episodes is not unusual.

THE HANGOVER HEADACHE

Naturally, some of you have never experienced a hangover headache, but others know all too well of its symptoms. The hangover headache may take a variety of forms. It is usually a throbbing, nagging pain that rudely reminds you of the indulgences of the night before. Though described for centuries the world over, the condition is not clearly understood. Alcohol, of course, plays an important role, but it may be the impurities in liquor more than the alcohol itself that are responsible for the headache. Some studies have shown that the hangover headache will not develop when sufficient quantities of *pure* ethyl alcohol, in contrast to liquor, are imbibed in a quiet and restful environment.

Hangover and its symptoms probably result from a combination of factors, among which are liquor, fatigue, smoke-filled rooms, altered sleeping hours, unusual or spicy foods—like exotic hors d'oeuvres—and perhaps a missed meal or two. Impurities in the various liquors (distillers keep the ingredients secret) and the biochemical products that are created in the body when liquor is metabolized are likely to play key roles.

There are many home remedies for the treatment of the hangover headache. Some respond to simple analgesics and others to antimigraine medications. The inhalation of oxygen may also be effective for some people. Recently, it has been suggested that aspirin or fruit sugar (fructose) taken before drinking may also exert some preventive influence on the development of the hangover headache. The most effective method of prevention, however, is obvious!

DYNAMITE WORKERS' HEADACHE

Nitrite compounds can cause pounding headaches resembling migraine. Because dynamite contains nitrites, workers in plants employing these compounds can suffer headaches caused by absorption of these substances through the skin. Regular exposure to these compounds may eventually result in tolerance to the substance, with a subsequent lessening of the headaches. However, vacations, long weekends, or other events or circumstances during which regular exposure is reduced may cause a recurrence of the headaches upon returning to work.

To avoid the re-exposure headache, dynamite workers have been known to place dynamite powder in their hatbands or elsewhere on their body so that exposure is maintained even while away from work. Protecting skin from direct contact while at work is also helpful.

The dynamite workers' headache is caused by the dilating effect of nitrites upon blood vessels. The headache is similar to the headache that occurs in persons taking nitroglycerin or other dilating substances for coronary heart disease or in some people after eating sandwich meats and hot dogs, which contain nitrite compounds for coloration. The "hot dog headache" and related disorders will be discussed further in Chapter 9.

SEX AND HEADACHE

Anyone who suffers from disabling headaches knows that "Not tonight, darling, I have a splitting headache" is not simply the ballad of the devious, frigid, or disinterested partner. Understandably, headache dulls the desire to participate in many activities, and sex is no exception.

It may be of some interest, however, that "Not tonight, darling, I'll *GET* a splitting headache" may also be a sincere plea of the headache sufferer. A severe headache can occur during intercourse and has been called benign orgasmic cephalalgia (cephal-, head; -algia, pain) because the discomfort most often occurs at the moment of orgasm. Benign orgasmic cephalalgia is more common in men, but women can also suffer from this condition.

Benign orgasmic cephalalgia usually occurs in individuals with migraine. The pain persists for moments to hours and is worsened by movement. Although the disorder itself is not usually serious, some potentially life-threatening conditions like stroke and bleeding into or around the brain may be heralded by headache occurring during sexual intercourse. Therefore, if a headache occurs during sexual activity, a thorough evaluation is necessary. This headache may represent a variation of the exertional headache.

Not long ago a sex therapist referred a twenty-two-year-old woman for evaluation. The young woman described how each sexual buildup was accompanied by a brutalizing headache that often forced her to cease her sexual activity. She stated that she had believed that her painful headache was "normal orgasm pain" and decided to see a sex therapist, since she did not enjoy sex because of this headache. Following a thorough evaluation, the woman was given antimigraine medication to take before intercourse and the orgasmic pain was prevented.

In the interest of preventive medicine, we note that studies on the association between sex and heart attacks and sex and strokes show that these catastrophic interruptions to sexual fulfillment are more likely to occur either during extramarital sexual activity or during endeavors with new partners. Somewhere in this there is a strong argument for fidelity!

Lest we end this section on these unhappy consequences of sexuality, we should mention that a few of our women patients have told us that having intercourse at the first sign of a migraine will prevent a severe headache from developing. This prompts us to offer yet another variation on the familiar phrase: "*Now*, darling, or I'll get a splitting headache!"

SUN AND HEADACHE

Although there is sufficient evidence to suggest that continued exposure to sunlight is harmful, vanity prevails and sunbathing remains popular. Headache is a prominent symptom in many who are exposed to the sun. The headache is often throbbing and may last for some time after exposure ceases. Wearing a hat while in the sun may help some of you.

Current evidence indicates that headache is one of the least important complications of frequent sun exposure. Cancer of the skin, premature wrinkling, and a variety of other medical conditions, including some serious blood disorders, are far better arguments against excessive sunbathing than is the development of headache.

The migraine triggered by the sun's glare is not the same problem as the headache from the heat of the sun beating down on your head. Wearing polarized lenses while in the sun may prevent the headache caused by flickering sunlight.

CONSTIPATION

Constipation can cause headaches. Considering that our diet suffers from an overabundance of refined foods and a poverty of bran and fibered substances, it is no wonder that so many individuals suffer from what advertisements so gently call "irregularity."

The headache associated with constipation does not have special characteristics, but a dull and throbbing headache is common. Other symptoms that can accompany constipation include nausea and lightheadedness. People who are depressed frequently suffer from constipation, and medication used for depression can worsen constipation.

The cause of the constipation headache is not known. Because constipation often occurs in people with a compulsive, migraine-type personality, and upon a background of emotional upset and depression, these factors may be important in causing the headache. One theory suggests that toxic substances from the stool are absorbed into the blood and are responsible for the headache. Another theory proposes that headaches come from the ballooning of the blocked intestine.

While the topic of constipation has some humorous connotations, current studies suggest that chronic constipation may provoke a variety of disorders of the gastrointestinal tract, including cancer, diverticulosis, and hemorrhoids. Eating whole wheat, bran, and other fibered foods and avoiding refined and processed carbohydrates, like white sugar, white bread, and white rice, may all help relieve constipation and lessen the risk of other conditions associated with it.

Chapter **8** The Diagnostic Evaluation, or
"The Work-Up"—What You Should Expect
from Your Doctor

The diagnostic evaluation, or "the work-up," is the investigation that a doctor undertakes to determine the basis for your symptoms. The manner in which a physician approaches your headache problem depends to a great extent upon the doctor's own medical training, philosophy, previous medical experiences, and the nature of his/her medical specialty. A medical evaluation of your problem can usually be divided into three parts: your medical history, a physical examination, and the investigative, or diagnostic, tests that are used to confirm or refute the physician's initial diagnosis.

YOUR MEDICAL HISTORY

Your medical history is a detailed account taken from you of the symptoms for which you are seeking medical help, together with a survey of various other important facets of your medical and social background. These are important in placing your current symptoms in perspective. Thus, the history-taking seeks out information about your present symptoms, past illnesses, allergies, family medical problems, and some details regarding the social circumstances in your life, such as your vocational interests, hobbies, alcohol and drug indulgences, and even strong food preferences or habits that are unusual.

When dealing with a headache problem, an accurate and complete description of the headache is the most valuable method of establishing a correct diagnosis. The more information that you provide, the more likely that a correct diagnosis will be made.

A complete and detailed history is important in the evaluation of any headache problem because many headache disorders have distinctive features that, when present, lead to a specific diagnosis. Because there are no visible signs associated with most headache conditions, the history is the only way that a correct diagnosis can be established. The physical examination and laboratory tests are likely to be normal in most patients suffering from just headaches.

Despite its importance, obtaining a detailed and accurate history is often very difficult. In order to elicit a good description of the headache problem and one that will help establish the correct diagnosis, the physician must ask the right questions and properly interpret the answers of the patient. The physician must also relate effectively to people of wide-ranging temperaments, intelligence, and eagerness to cooperate.

However, gathering the necessary information during history-taking is not simply a matter of asking the appropriate questions and listing the answers. Even if the doctor does make the necessary inquiries, individuals vary considerably in their ability and willingness to give accurate and detailed information. Some patients are unable to remember important facts or ignore what seem to them to be trivial or coincidental incidents or events. Others are incapable of expressing the information in an understandable manner; vocabularies and verbal ability vary. Sometimes the necessary interruption of a patient's story or description will make him/her quite irritable, so that further information or responses to questions are delivered in a defensive and abbreviated manner. Evasive, rambling, and confused responses make the effort at history-taking even more arduous. These elements all add to the difficulty of headache diagnosis.

A problem that the doctor commonly encounters during the taking of a history is the vast difference in the way individuals describe the same symptoms. For example, an uncomfortable feeling in the head may be characterized as

a boring pain,
a piercing sharpness,
a heaviness, or
a dull ache.

Out-of-focus vision may be explained as

a blurriness,
a dizziness of the eyes, or
a blindness.

Properly interpreting these varied descriptions of the same symptom is often quite difficult yet critical in establishing a correct diagnosis.

Doctors often find that taking a reliable medical history is further complicated by the biases created by media descriptions of headaches, such as in magazine articles, on television shows, and by advertisers offering cures that are frequently at variance with accepted medical knowledge.

Many people go to their doctors convinced that their headaches are due to specific disorders, ranging from sinus problems to brain tumors, and quite often there is no valid basis for such beliefs. A self-diagnosis based on a dramatization of a hospital scene or on a sixty-second commercial seems very attractive to many people.

Accurate media presentations can serve an important educational role. Some patients have been alerted to important medical conditions and symptoms by television shows, and most producers of these dramas strive for realistic presentations. But, unfortunately, the complexities of disease preclude a single case presentation on a television show from covering the many exceptions and variations of human illness. So while accurate medical entertainment may have some beneficial value, it may give others false assurance or undue concern.

A few years ago a thirty-year-old woman was evaluated for the complaint of weakness, so severe that she could barely stand without assistance. She stated that she was a "soap opera addict," and she had "suffered" many of the diseases dramatized on the serials. She assumed that her present illness was just another "TV disease." Unhappily, this woman really did suffer from an incurable disease. She died within months of her first being seen.

Physicians themselves may also contribute to a misunderstanding of proper medical care, which ultimately leads to poor communication between doctor and patient. For example, over the years some doctors have routinely administered penicillin or other antibiotics to most patients with a sore throat, even though antibiotics are not usually required. Overuse of antibiotics diminishes the effectiveness of some of these drugs and if used in the wrong setting, may actually make a condition worse. But now, ironically, the physician who refuses to administer penicillin to someone with a sore throat may be greeted with hostility if the patient has been led to believe that routine administration of antibiotics is good medical practice.

While taking a medical history, the physician will make observations about your personality and temperament, how you react to suggestions, and your ability to express yourself. For example, some patients fidget, wring their hands, or cry while they give their history. Some patients will show great concern and anxiety while detailing mild and infrequent symptoms, whereas others will appear indifferent while describing severely painful, frequent, and even disabling symptoms. If observed and interpreted correctly, individual personality traits will help your physician diagnose your problems and plan a treatment to meet your individual needs.

Following are the basic elements of a good medical history for headache:

General Profile

Age.
Occupation.
Have you had other medical illnesses?
Do you have any allergies to medicines or drugs?
What do you do for fun, relaxation, amusement?
What do you do for work?

Do you have a normal sleep pattern (sleep usually six to eight hours a night)?

As a child, do you remember your family as being excitable or calm?

Does anyone else in your family suffer from headaches? (It is common for several members of the same family to suffer from migraine headaches.)

What are your hobbies?

Do you have any unusual habits or routines that expose you to chemicals or other toxic substances?

Do you eat or drink any unusual foods?

Do you eat or drink large amounts of any one food or beverage?

Do you consider yourself a generally happy person?

Are you usually calm and content?

Are you often bored and restless?

How many members are in your family?

Does your present family have a specific personality?

What is your current life-style?

Do you often worry about money?

Do you sometimes worry without having any specific reason?

Do you ever feel anxious for no reason?

These questions are important because your level of happiness and the many emotional and social factors that can promote, aggravate, or alleviate headache must be determined.

Details of Your Headaches—Some people have more than one type of headache and detailing the characteristics of each type is of great importance since the treatment of different types of headaches can vary greatly. Following are some of the questions that your doctor should raise:

ONSET: It is very important to understand when and under what circumstances each of your different headaches first occurred.

At what age did they first begin?

Was any particular event associated with their onset, such as menstruation or pregnancy?

Did the initial headache begin during or following a period of great emotional stress or frustration?
Did they occur during or after physical activity?
Was illness associated with the onset?

PATTERN AND FREQUENCY:

Do your headaches occur about once a month, weekly, or three or four times a day?
Are your headaches predictable? In other words, do you have a warning?
Are your headaches worse during some months or seasons?
Has the pattern changed over the years? In what way?
Do your headaches have a relationship to meals?
Do your headaches happen at one special time of day?
Do your headaches occur only at special times or during weekends or vacations?

DURATION: Some headaches last for specific lengths of time. Determining the duration of an average attack can be very useful in diagnosing a headache. A migraine headache may last up to four or five days, but a cluster headache typically begins and ends within fifteen to forty-five minutes. Occasionally, the intensity of a headache episode varies considerably from beginning to end. All this information must be shared with your physician, and you should be aware of your own headache pattern. Self-knowledge is often the first step in headache alleviation.

NATURE AND LOCATION OF THE PAIN: How would you best describe your pain? Is it

dull,
throbbing,
piercing,
squeezing,
crushing,
boring,
burning?

(Recently a patient gruesomely likened her pain behind an eye to that of a sharpened pencil being pushed slowly through her eyeball. This is not an uncommon description.)

Where does it hurt you?
Does your pain alternate from side to side or remain well localized to a single region?
Does it radiate from the neck forward and wrap around your head as though you were wearing a hat many sizes too small?
Does it feel as though a hammer were pounding at your temples?
Are your headaches incapacitating?
Are your headaches interfering or annoying but allow you to function during them?

RELIEF:

What efforts have you found successful in reducing your pain? Resting in a dark room? Inducing vomiting? Pacing? Running?
Do you preoccupy yourself during a headache?
Do you seek inactivity and solitude?
Have you found that ice packs help?
Does application of heat help?
Does assuming a particular position help, such as lowering or raising your head?
Does drinking tea or coffee help?
What medications have you taken for your headaches and which ones have helped?
Is there anything that tends to make your headache worse?

ASSOCIATED SYMPTOMS: Many additional symptoms can occur along with your headache. The presence of visual disturbances, such as flickering spots, blurriness, and double or decreased vision, that lead to or are present with your headache is very important.

Is there a sensitivity to light (photophobia) or discomfort from sounds (hyperacusis) during your headaches?
Do you notice the presence of tingling in any part of the body? Numbness? Weakness? Dizziness? Nausea? Diarrhea? Fever? Stiff neck?

Does an impairment of word expression ever occur?
Does an impairment of memory occur?

TRIGGERING EVENTS: Activities, foods, emotional disturbances, or other events can precipitate headaches in many people.

Does your headache develop following or during sleep? Exertion? Fatigue?
Do you get headaches when you are very tired?
Do you notice your headache linked with eating or drinking coffee? Hot dogs? Ice Cream? Alcohol? Chinese food? Other beverages or foods?
Does any medication provoke a headache?
Are your headaches related to periods of hunger or long intervals between meals?
Do glaring or flickering lights from a poor television picture or sunlight coming through the trees during an afternoon's drive provoke your headaches?
Do changes in air temperature, barometric pressure, or damp, rainy days bring on headaches?
Does sudden exposure to cold seem to have any influence on your headache problem?
Is your furnace working properly?
Are hormonal changes, such as menstruation or ovulation, associated with your headaches?

After a complete medical history has been obtained, the diagnostic evaluation enters the next step: the physical examination. Your doctor may think of additional questions or you may remember more details or symptoms during the course of the work-up, so the history-taking actually continues throughout the entire doctor-patient interaction.

Very often these details are not easily recalled, and important patterns are thus not recognized. The following is a headache chart which can record headaches for a weekly period. Each chart will indicate the number of headaches occurring that week. A review of your charts can sometimes reveal distinct headache patterns.

WEEKLY HEADACHE DIARY

NAME
WEEK of

Day/Date	Time of Onset	Severity	Location of Pain	Events Preceding Onset
MON.				
TUES.				
WEDS.				
THURS.				
FRI.				
SAT.				
SUN.				

Severity	*Degree of Relief* (Examples)
1–Annoying	Slight
2–Troublesome	Moderate
3–Moderately severe	Complete
4–Quite severe	
5–Incapacitating	

Triggers	Drugs (Dose)	Other Actions Taken	Degree of Relief	Time of Maximum Relief

Triggers (Examples)
   Emotions (e.g., frustration, anger, elation, anxiety)
   Foods (name)
   Physical exertion
   Menstrual period
   Weather change
   Missed meals
   Letdown after stress
   Weekend
   Holiday or vacation
   Extra sleep
   (Others)

THE PHYSICAL EXAMINATION

Nearly everyone has undergone a routine physical examination. A "general checkup" is designed to survey the major body systems. When headache symptoms are present, a more detailed evaluation is very important.

A neurological examination tests the functions of the brain, spinal cord, nerves, and muscles. Therefore, in a neurological examination, mental processes, motor abilities, and sensory responses—such as sight, hearing, and feeling—are evaluated.

The Mental Status Examination—The test of mental function is performed by requiring you to carry out certain mental tasks, the successful completion of which suggests a normal functioning of certain areas of the brain. Memory, orientation, calculation, judgment, and reasoning are frequently surveyed.

The examination of mental status is not a psychiatric evaluation, but frequently when this portion of the examination begins, some individuals incorrectly become concerned that their doctor believes that the headache is of psychological origin.

The mental examination often begins by testing basic orientation. This is done by asking your name, birth date, the current month, and your present whereabouts. To further test your memory, you may be asked to name the presidents of the United States in reverse order, or some other question that requires recall of specific facts, but juxtaposed in a new way. You are not expected to recall all the presidents, and the interpretation of this test by the doctor takes into account your age, education, and general background.

Because the regions of the brain responsible for recent memory, what has happened in the last few hours or days, may differ from those for past memory—for example, remembering the presidents' names—you may be given a short list of ordinary items, such as a balloon, a ribbon, and a flashlight, and then be asked to name them a few moments later. Remembering a short list of numbers and recalling a simple story are also methods used to test recent memory.

The ability to think abstractly is sometimes evaluated by asking you to interpret well-known proverbs. What do people mean when they say:

"A stitch in time saves nine"?
"A bird in the hand is worth two in the bush"?
"Don't cry over spilled milk"?
"People who live in glass houses shouldn't throw stones"?

Ideally, the responses will reflect an interpretive quality rather than a simple concrete understanding of the words alone. For example, to the proverb "Don't cry over spilled milk," it would be appropriate to state that one should not worry over events that have already occurred. A concrete response would be "You shouldn't cry if the milk is spilled."

The value of proverb interpretation, as with other parts of the mental status test, is limited by many factors, including basic intelligence and cultural background. Recently, a medical student expressed concern about a patient whose mental status examination reflected an inability to interpret proverbs. The patient, although able to speak English quite well, had immigrated to this country only a year before taking the test. The proverb test, in this instance, had no value because of the patient's relative unfamiliarity with the new language, its nuances, and its idioms.

Ability to perform mathematical calculations can be tested by asking you to mentally compute. One common method is to require you to start at one hundred and subtract by various numbers.

Many other methods can be used to evaluate mental functions. Some people consider these exercises ludicrously simple, and some think they are frightfully difficult. It should be comforting to know that we all differ considerably in our ability to perform such mental tasks, and as we have already suggested, performance depends upon your education, your level of anxiety or depression, and many other important factors that must be taken into account in the final interpretation of your mental performance.

The Examination of Cranial Nerve Function—The cranial nerves are twelve paired nerves that emerge from the lower part of the brain. They are responsible for smell, vision, taste, hearing, face and jaw movements, swallowing, articulation, and most sensations about the face. The cranial nerve examination evaluates these functions.

This portion of the examination is particularly important to an individual with headaches because disorders of the head and neck that cause head pain, such as tumors, may directly or indirectly affect the cranial nerves. Pain can be referred through nerves to a location distant from its sources, so that pain originating inside the head may be "referred" elsewhere around the head or face, possibly to the forehead, eye, or behind an ear.

The Motor Examination—The motor examination consists of testing strength and coordination. It includes looking for wasting muscles and abnormal movements, such as tremors, and also checking muscle reflexes, such as the knee reflex, by tapping various muscle tendons.

The reflex examination usually provides information about the anatomical communications between the brain, spinal cord, nerves, and muscles. These reflexes, contrary to popular misunderstanding, are not the same as "reaction reflexes," like slamming on the brakes of an automobile to avoid an impending accident.

Coordination is tested in various ways. It can be evaluated in the arms by having you touch your nose with a fingertip or perform a skillful movement like writing. In the legs, coordination can be tested by having you rapidly tap a foot on the floor or run the heel of one foot down the opposite shin. Coordination, balance, and muscle strength can be evaluated effectively by simply observing you as you walk.

The Sensory Examination—This examination evaluates your reaction to various stimuli. We can test your reaction to pain by pricking your skin lightly with a pin. Your ability to sense tactile sensations is tested by stroking your skin with cotton. Vibration sensation is tested by applying a tuning fork to your wrists and ankles. Your ability to sense position is tested by wriggling one of your toes or fingers up and down and asking in what direction it is pointing.

An additional sensory function is tested by asking you to close your eyes and identify an object placed in your hand or to name numerals or letters as they are written on your skin.

The performance of every patient must be interpreted by taking into consideration many factors, including information from the medical history, the ability to understand and cooperate in the testing, and the impact that emotional states or moods, like depression or anxiety, may have upon your performance. To interpret, rather than simply record, subtle inconsistencies and abnormalities is one of the most difficult challenges in practicing medicine.

Following the medical history and the physical examination, you and your physician should discuss your symptoms and his/her findings. The doctor should allow ample time for you to ask questions and express doubts or other feelings, including your concerns and fears regarding your illness. Your doctor must also explain his/her diagnostic intentions and what treatment methods will be employed. When you leave the physician's office, you should feel that you were carefully examined, had an opportunity to fully express yourself, and have a good idea of how the doctor is going to approach your headache problem.

THE INVESTIGATIVE TESTS

To help substantiate or refute your physician's impressions, some further tests will usually be ordered. The choice of which procedures to perform is determined by the information gathered from the medical history and the physical examination, and your physician's judgment.

Investigative studies can be divided into *noninvasive* and *invasive* types. Noninvasive tests do not require entrance into the body, and there is usually little or no pain or risk involved. Routine X rays, for example, are considered noninvasive, although they do expose you to some radiation and should never be performed unless they are absolutely necessary.

Invasive tests vary in their likelihood of causing complications and associated discomfort. Taking blood is an invasive procedure but only mildly painful and carrying only a minimal risk. However, an arteriogram, described on page 186, may cause serious complications. Ideally, your physician will order only those tests essential for an accurate evaluation and order them in sequence of increasing risk, attempting if at all possible to establish the diagnosis with noninvasive procedures.

The following are some of the procedures that your doctor may order. Some of them, particularly the invasive ones, are not routinely employed in most headache problems. You should ask your physician to explain why the tests are being ordered and what risks are involved.

Blood Tests—A series of blood and urine tests is frequently ordered. The tests survey for various medical problems, some of which may contribute to the headaches.

X Rays—Skull and neck X rays are also frequently ordered. Skull X rays may show abnormal deposits of calcium that can accompany tumors, infections, or blood vessel abnormalities. The X rays may also show evidence of previous skull injury or skull deformities. X rays of the neck can show arthritis, fractures, or other abnormalities, any of which could be the origin of headache.

Because radiation can have harmful effects on a fetus, women should avoid X rays if even a remote chance of pregnancy exists. All premenopausal women who engage in sexual intercourse without the use of contraceptive measures should consider themselves potentially pregnant. Therefore, routine X rays should be taken only during the first ten days of the menstrual cycle. Of course, if there is some extraordinary reason for X rays, then the risks must be weighed against the need for them. In all instances, protective lead shielding should be used.

Electroencephalogram (EEG)—Electroencephalography is often a valuable test in evaluating headaches. The EEG is a study of the brain's functioning as reflected by electrical patterns that are converted and amplified by the machine to a pattern that is recorded on moving paper. Special electrodes are pasted to the scalp to detect the electrical activity of the brain through the skull (see Photos 1 and 2, page 93).

The EEG is painless and safe. Contrary to the concern of some people, an EEG records the brain's activity but does not allow anyone to read your mind.

Brain Scan—A brain scan is also painless and relatively safe, but does require an injection into the bloodstream of a substance that contains slight radioactivity. Brain scanning is based upon the principle that when very small amounts of a certain radioactive substance are injected into the bloodstream, they will enter brain tissue. With the use of a machine similar to a Geiger counter, the pattern of absorption of this radioactive substance by various areas of the brain can be determined (Photos 3 and 4, page 94). In certain abnormal conditions, such as brain tumors and strokes, the abnormal tissue may absorb more or less of the radioactive substance than the surrounding normal tissue. This test should not be performed in pregnant or possibly pregnant women.

CAT (Computerized Axial Tomography) Scan, or EMI Scan—Recent scientific developments have resulted in an advanced investigative technique known as computerized axial tomography (CAT), or EMI scanning. EMI refers to one of the manufacturers of this unit—the European Musical Instrument Company. This test is usually noninvasive. It uses a very complex computerized X ray-technique to "photograph" brain tissue. This is accomplished with the use of a large device, part of which rotates around the head and photographically records the brain from different positions (Photo 5, page 95). These picture slices can be displayed as photographs for evaluation (Photo 6, page 95).

The CAT scan is painless and relatively safe, but some radiation exposure does occur. Also, the injection into the bloodstream of a special substance can enhance the test's accuracy, but this makes it an invasive procedure. With some machines the degree of radiation exposure is no more than that encountered with conventional skull X rays.

CAT scanning has made a great contribution to medicine and

has made possible the diagnosis of many neurological conditions that previously could be confirmed only by invasive procedures. This test is presently very expensive to perform.

Cerebral Arteriography (Angiography)—A cerebral arteriogram is a study of brain blood vessels. It is an invasive procedure and should generally not be used for investigating headache conditions unless abnormalities have been suggested by preliminary studies. The test is performed by first injecting into the bloodstream a material known as a *contrast medium.* This material, commonly but incorrectly called a dye, contrasts against other brain tissue, and the blood vessels containing the substance stand out and can be seen when the head is X-rayed. Because the normal pattern of the cerebral blood vessels is known, any variations can be spotted (Photo 7, page 95).

The arteriogram is important in evaluating certain neurological conditions: brain tumors, blood clots, and blood vessel abnormalities. Although the test causes only minimal discomfort, there are some serious risks, including the possibility of inducing a stroke, particularly in elderly patients.

Lumbar Puncture—The lumbar puncture, also called a spinal tap, is performed by inserting a needle between two vertebrae in the lower back. When the needle enters the space around the spinal cord, the spinal fluid will flow through the needle, allowing measurement of the fluid pressure and collection of the fluid for evaluation. The spinal fluid is a clear water-like substance produced by blood vessels and cells in the brain. The spinal fluid nourishes, bathes, and cushions the brain and the spinal cord. Certain abnormalities of the nervous system can be detected through changes in the spinal fluid.

Although the lumbar puncture is an invasive test, the actual procedure causes only minimal discomfort. Some people undergoing this test will experience an uncomfortable but not serious headache a few hours after the test. Many physicians prefer not to perform a lumbar puncture in the evaluation of routine headache problems. Although under most circumstances the procedure carries little risk, it must not be done in certain medical situations.

The Pneumoencephalogram—The pneumoencephalogram, like the arteriogram, is a contrast procedure, but this test uses air rather than a chemical for contrast. It is done by first performing a lumbar puncture while the patient is seated in a special tilting chair. Air is pushed through the needle, and as it bubbles upward, it encircles the brain and enters the large fluid-filled channels of the brain (the ventricles). X rays are then performed, and the ventricles and surrounding spaces, now filled with air, can be seen.

This invasive test is associated with some risk and is moderately painful, often producing headache, nausea, and vomiting, which can last longer than a day. A pneumoencephalogram is not ordinarily performed in the evaluation of most headache problems. Like the arteriogram, it should not be routinely performed.

By now you should be able to see that taking a medical history, accurately interpreting the results of the physical examination, and deciding which tests, if any, must be ordered and which can be delayed required good judgment on the part of the physician. Because wise judgments are so vital to the practice of good medicine, we think that it would be appropriate to offer an observation regarding malpractice suits and the practice of defensive medicine.

Defensive medicine means the use of tests which *might* be considered unnecessary in a particular medical situation but which are performed, nevertheless, so the physician cannot be accused of overlooking something that, in retrospect, was important.

A physician must always weigh the potential value of a diagnostic test or treatment against the possible adverse reactions and risks. During the work-up, if, in the judgment of a physician, a diagnosis appears relatively well established without resorting to invasive investigations, the physician may choose not to order these tests, or at least delay them. This, of course, requires good medical judgment. If a physician is competent, these judgments will, over the years, spare countless patients the risks, discomfort, and cost of excessive testing.

But during the lifetime of a physician who may see thousands of patients and many variations of diseases, instances may occur when the unusual and unexpected happens. In such circumstances, these special tests, in retrospect, could have established a diagnosis earlier if they had not been delayed. Even the wisest and most competent physician will eventually find himself or herself in such a circumstance if restraint has been used over the years in ordering what appeared to be unnecessary tests. The point, of course, is that any single instance of misjudgment makes that physician vulnerable to a malpractice suit.

Some malpractice suits are justifiable, but others are not. A lifetime of giving qualified, conscientious, and cautious medical care to thousands can be destroyed by the implications arising from one exceptional event. The fear of this possibility has forced many doctors to practice defensive medicine. A large part of the risk and the cost of modern medical care reflects this decision.

There is no easy solution to the problem. Responsible members of the medical and legal professions and representatives of the general public must establish reasonable guidelines. There is really no acceptable defense for the practice of careless and bad medicine, but the complexities inherent in delivering medical care must be taken into account. Restraint within the legal profession, education of the medical consumer, and an aggressive weeding out of unqualified practitioners of medicine seem to be the critical steps necessary to achieve a solution to this problem.

Chapter 9 Headaches and the Foods You Eat

Few matters related to health have received as much attention and stirred as much controversy and debate as the subject of diet and its influence on our health. Most headaches do not appear to be influenced by dietary considerations, but some foods do appear to provoke headaches in some people. The relationship between foods and headache is not well understood and disagreement exists even among headache authorities. Complicating our ability to understand this issue is a person's apparent changing sensitivity to possible headache-provoking foods. Thus, some foods potentially capable of provoking a headache may appear to do so only under certain biological circumstances—say, during the menstrual period—while at other times the same food substance will not cause a headache. Because of this cyclical or intermittent sensitivity, plus the likelihood that headache sufferers differ in their vulnerability, it is quite difficult to identify with certainty those foods capable of provoking headaches.

Four major substances in particular have been implicated.

THE CAFFEINE HEADACHE

In earlier chapters we pointed out that caffeine has a number of important properties, among them its ability to constrict blood vessels and to act as a stimulant to the heart and the brain. Caffeine can also raise blood sugar, stimulate urine production, and perhaps assist in the absorption of medication from the stomach.

The history of caffeine is old, and anecdotes regarding caffeine add perspective to our current use of this substance. About 850 A.D., an Arabian shepherd observed strange behavior in his flock after the animals had eaten some berries. The shepherd decided to try some of the berries and, we are told, that shepherd enjoyed the first "coffee break."

It is also alleged that a Chinese Buddhist fell asleep during a nine-year meditation. In despair, he is alleged to have cut off his eyelashes. The eyelashes fell to the ground and, as the story goes, sprouted caffeinated tea.

The Arabians used caffeine as a stimulant to remain alert during long religious services. By the seventeenth century the drink had been introduced in England, and coffeehouses in London became the centers of social and political activity. Today, coffee and other caffeine-containing foods and beverages are so much a part of social and dietary structure they have become part of our way of life. The morning and afternoon tea and the coffee break are considered part of the rights of employees. We go on coffee dates and attend coffee klatches. We eat coffee cakes off coffee tables in coffeehouses or coffee shops while, perhaps, in the background is the music of "Tea for Two" or "Java Jive." In 1732 Bach wrote "Coffee Cantata" in response to Frederick the Great's suggested ban on caffeine.

Whether caffeine is "the devil's brew," a "loathsome poison," or "the nectar of the gods," as it is claimed by some, a large variety of foods and medications contain caffeine. Here are the amounts of caffeine * in some common foods:

* Determinations by Dr. Alan J. Burg, Cambridge, Massachusetts, in Manber, op. cit.

Coffee per cup
Brewed, 80–120 mg.
Instant, 66–100 mg.
Tea per cup
Leaf, 30–75 mg.
Bag, 42–100 mg.
Instant, 30–60 mg.
Cocoa per cup
Up to 50 mg.
Cola per 8-ounce glass
15–30 mg.
Chocolate bar
25 mg.

Coffee is the main source of caffeine for most of the adult population, and it is estimated that two and one-half billion pounds of coffee are consumed annually in the United States. The average coffee drinker drinks more than two cups each day, and almost one-half of coffee drinkers surveyed admitted that drinking coffee is not simply an enjoyable indulgence but actually a habit. More than one-half said that they felt the need for it in the morning, and without coffee they just don't feel well.†

Foods and beverages are not the only sources of caffeine. Besides coffee, tea, cola, and chocolate, substantial amounts of caffeine are in many medications. Among the more popular brand-name medications that contain caffeine are Anacin, Fiorinal, Cafergot, Darvon Compound, Excedrin, Vanquish, and most sinus headache preparations. Many of these products are taken in abusive dosages, and when the daily caffeine intake from all sources is tabulated, the total is astounding.

The symptoms of caffeinism can be divided into mood disturbances, sleep disturbances, and withdrawal symptoms. The mood disturbances may take the form of anxiety symptoms, such as tremor, agitation, muscle twitching, palpitations, gastrointestinal

† A. Goldstein, S. Kaizer, and O. Whitby, "Psychotropic Effects of Caffeine in Man. IV: Quantitative and Qualitative Differences Associated with Habituation to Coffee," in *Clinical Pharmacology and Therapeutics*, Vol. 10, No. 489 (July–August 1969), p. 489.

distress, lightheadedness, and headaches. The sleep disturbances may include delayed onset and more frequent awakenings.

Withdrawal symptoms may occur following excessive intake, and headaches can be one of them. Large amounts of caffeine taken during the day are likely to cause significant withdrawal symptoms during the night. Such patients tend to awaken in the morning with a headache and grogginess that are generally not reversed until they ingest one or two cups of coffee, along with several caffeine-containing tablets. While there are many other causes for morning headaches, we believe that excessive caffeine ingestion must be considered to be an important possibility.

Many of our headache patients have consumed incredibly large amounts of caffeine and quite probably suffered a number of severe headaches as a result. One particular patient stands out in this respect: He drank approximately fifteen cups of coffee daily. In addition, he habitually had at least three or four bottles of a cola beverage and four chocolate bars, and because he had daily headaches, he also took a variety of caffeine-containing drugs, including Anacin, Fiorinal, and Excedrin. In addition to headaches, his symptoms included tremulousness, nervousness, palpitations, and a personality change as well as unexplained weight loss. His most painful bouts of headache were in the early-morning hours, many hours after his last dose of caffeine was taken. We conjectured that caffeine withdrawal accounted for many of his morning headache attacks, and his afternoon headaches and other symptoms were in part due to abusive amounts of caffeine. His treatment consisted of carefully and slowly discontinuing the amount of caffeine ingested. After a short time, significant improvement in the patient's headache symptoms was noticed, and although some headaches remained, they responded to conventional therapy.

Our understanding of the immense influence of caffeine has been aided by a report by Dr. John Greden, who studied a series of patients suffering symptoms of anxiety, insomnia, and dizziness.* The people in the test were initially diagnosed as having anxiety neurosis, but Dr. Greden showed that all of the patients were

---

* J. Greden, "Anxiety or Caffeinism: A Diagnostic Dilemma," in *American Journal of Psychiatry* (Oct. 1974), p. 1089.

suffering from caffeine intoxication. After restricting their use of caffeine-containing substances, they improved dramatically.

While this important contribution to our understanding of caffeine and our behavior must not be taken lightly, do not overestimate its implications either. Most people who are nervous and tense are probably not suffering from caffeine intoxication. But if you are experiencing headaches, particularly when elements of nervousness are present, you should carefully consider your intake of cola drinks, chocolate, tea, coffee, and other caffeine-containing foods and medications. Cola, incidentally, is likely to be the single largest source of caffeine in the adolescent population, and like other caffeinated items, it is somewhat addictive.

Before leaving the subject of caffeine, we must comment on a potential hazard related to the use of decaffeinated coffee. Our discussion might motivate some of you to use this alternative to coffee. While decaffeinated coffee is very low in caffeine content, the decaffeinating process uses special chemicals to remove the caffeine. Some of these chemicals have been shown to cause cancer in experimental animals. A major food processor that produces Sanka and Brim has recently discontinued, after considerable governmental and consumer-group pressure, its use of the chemical trichlorethylene in the decaffeinating process (trichlorethylene is also used for dry cleaning, spot removing, air freshening, and as a degreasing agent). This food processor is now decaffeinating coffee with another chemical, and the safety of this alternative process is currently being studied.

AMINES IN YOUR FOOD

Throughout this book we have mentioned the importance of substances called amines (see Appendix). The amines play a very important role in normal brain function as well as in general physiology. The body manufactures from items in the diet most of the amines that it needs. When the body's normal production or level of amines is altered, emotional as well as physical disease, including depression, mania, migraine, and Parkinson's disease, may result.

A large number of everyday food items contains amines, and it is generally believed that headaches may result in some people after eating foods containing unusually high levels of these substances. Below is a list of some of the food items that contain one or more of the amines.

Cheeses (except cottage cheese and cream cheese)
Vinegar or food containing vinegar (relishes, pickled items, catsup, prepared mustard, mayonnaise, salad dressings, Worcestershire sauce, chili sauce, steak sauces)
Game meats
Liver, kidneys, sweetbreads, brains, other organ meats
Pickled herring, caviar, preserved fish
Alcoholic beverages (beer, wine [particularly sherry, Chianti, red]), desserts containing alcohol
Chocolate
Cream, sour cream, yogurt
Foods containing yeast extracts (Found in some prepared soups, bouillon cubes, and other items. Learn from labels.)
Fruits and vegetables
    Spinach
    Citrus fruits (particularly oranges)
    Bananas
    Figs, plums
    Pineapples
    Raisins
    Avocados
    Broad beans (lima, soybeans, etc.)
    Onions
Miscellaneous
    All protein food in which aging or breakdown is used to enhance flavor (smoked, aged)
Pork

Undoubtedly many of you who suffer from headaches will find that you regularly eat a number of the foods listed above. We caution that your headaches do not necessarily result from these foods. However, if large quantities of one item are eaten, if one or more of these substances are consistently part of your diet, or if your headaches seem to occur soon after eating any one or more of these foods, it seems reasonable to restrict them in your diet in order to see whether this makes a positive difference. If you do improve, then you should continue restricting the foods to determine with certainty that your improvement was not simply coincidental.

Then you can double-check how these foods affect you by returning one item at a time to your diet. Perhaps you will be able to isolate which food or foods are responsible for your symptoms. Keep in mind, however, that it may be the total quantity of amines ingested rather than the amines that come from any one substance that is aggravating your headache problem.

Whether these foods and beverages do actually provoke headaches remains a controversial issue and many medical investigators disagree on this subject, so it would be wise to regard these items simply as potential triggers to painful headache. Several of our patients seem consistently sensitive to these substances. Chocolate, fatty foods, and citrus fruits (particularly oranges) are most often cited by patients who believe that their headaches occur regularly after eating one or more of these items.

Alcohol is particularly likely to be the guilty agent. You may remember that alcohol dilates the blood vessels, and it also contains varying amounts of amines, including histamine. Wine contains abundant amounts of histamine, and red wine contains more of the amine than does white wine.

THE CHINESE RESTAURANT SYNDROME AND MONOSODIUM GLUTAMATE (MSG)

Chinese-style cooking is popular throughout the world, but for some years it has been apparent that many individuals simply cannot eat Chinese cooking without becoming sick. A few years ago a condition called the "Chinese restaurant syndrome" was described. This syndrome embraces a variety of symptoms, including headache, sweating, and tightness and burning in the chest, face, jaw, and body trunk. These bizarre symptoms usually occur within fifteen to twenty-five minutes after eating Chinese food.

"The Chinese restaurant syndrome" was first recognized by Dr. Herbert Schaumberg of New York. Dr. Schaumberg, a Chinese food enthusiast, began an investigation of the numerous unpleasant sensations he experienced after eating Chinese food. First, he looked into the possibility of contamination and found none. He then undertook an effort, together with the chef at his favorite restaurant, to identify which among the various substances that he ate was responsible for the symptoms. By the process of elimination, he concluded that the food additive and flavor enhancer monosodium glutamate (MSG) was the agent that provoked what he called "the Chinese restaurant syndrome."

The syndrome occurs in certain vulnerable individuals who suffer a variety of unpleasant sensations following the eating of food containing MSG, particularly on an empty stomach. It is believed by some authorities that most patients who suffer from the syndrome are apparently unable to properly metabolize MSG and therefore experience a rapid build-up in the bloodstream following ingestion. It is this rapid build-up that allegedly provokes the symptoms. When food not containing MSG is ingested *prior* to MSG-containing substances, MSG absorption is delayed and the build-up in the bloodstream occurs more slowly. Thus symptoms may not develop.

The issue of monosodium glutamate and its adverse effects goes beyond eating in Chinese restaurants. Approximately twenty thousand tons of MSG are used yearly in the United States. This substance appears in a wide variety of packaged and processed foods and beverages. MSG is used to enhance food flavor but has no known nutritional value. Presently, there is interest in the possible hazards of MSG consumption, including brain abnormalities in young experimental animals. Recently MSG was ordered removed from all commercially prepared baby foods. In addition to causing the symptoms of the Chinese restaurant syndrome and possibly affecting the developing brain, monosodium glutamate may have an adverse effect on heart rhythm in some

---

° H. H. Schaumberg and R. Byck, "Sin Cib-Syn: Accent on Glutamate," in *New England Journal of Medicine* (July 1968), p. 105.

people,† cause shuddering or shivering attacks in children,‡ and cause additional adverse symptoms§ in adults.

The connection between headaches and MSG is important; it is estimated that 10 to 25 percent of the population may be sensitive to MSG and suffer from its effects. In some, headaches may be the only symptom associated with MSG sensitivity.

It has been shown that MSG-induced headaches are very similar to migraine or muscle contraction headaches.* The headaches are characterized by pounding pain over the temples and a tightness around the forehead. The pain tends to occur within twenty to thirty minutes following the ingestion of food containing MSG, particularly when eaten on an empty stomach.

Monosodium glutamate is often found in the following items. This is not a complete list.

Instant soups
Canned soups
Dry-roasted nuts
Processed meats
Self-basting turkeys
Some potato chip products
Instant gravies
Many TV dinners
Packaged tenderizers and seasonings (Aćcent, Lawry's Seasoned Salt, etc.)

People who notice a headache after eating should attempt to determine whether or not MSG was present in the items that they ingested. This, of course, requires a careful reading of all food labels, a habit that all consumers should develop. If it appears

† H. H. Neumann, "Soup? It May Be Hazardous to Your Health," in *American Heart Journal* (August 1976), p. 267.

‡ L. Reif-Lehrer and M. G. Stemmermann, "Monosodium Glutamate in Children (Correspondence)," in *New England Journal of Medicine* (Dec. 1975), p. 1204.

§ L. Reif-Lehrer, "Possible Significance of Adverse Reactions to Glutamate in Humans," in *Federation Proceedings*, Vol. 35 (Sept. 1976), pp. 2205–11.

* H. H. Schaumberg, R. Byck, R. Gerstl, and J. H. Mashman, "Monosodium L-Glutamate: Its Pharmacology and Role in the Chinese Restaurant Syndrome," in *Science* (Feb. 1969), p. 163.

likely that your headaches are due to MSG, then elimination of all sources of this substance from your diet seems wise.

NITRITES AND THE HOT DOG HEADACHE

Do you ever suffer a pounding headache after eating a hot dog or a processed-meat sandwich? Probably the meat contains nitrites. This headache condition has been called the "hot dog headache" and results from the dilation of blood vessels. The nitrite compounds contained in many of these food items cause the vascular dilation. You will recall that nitrite compounds, like the nitroglycerin used for treatment in heart attacks and heart pain, and the nitrites absorbed through the skin of dynamite workers, can sometimes induce headaches.

Nitrite has been used for centuries as a meat preservative. Its use by the early Romans is recorded: it was used in a brine for curing meat.

It is estimated that more than twelve billion pounds of nitrite substances are annually added to our food supply.* These compounds are used to give meat a special cured taste, to add color— red or pink—and to act in preventing botulism food poisoning, which is potentially fatal.

Among the foods that may contain the nitrites are:

Canned hams
Corned beef
Hot dogs
Salami
Bologna
Sausage
Bacon
Peperoni
Smoked fish

There is presently an investigation into the safety of using nitrite substances in food. The concern goes beyond the issue of

* *Consumer Reports* (March 1976). p. 127.

headaches. Nitrite substances have a tendency to combine with some amines to form compounds called nitrosamines. The nitrosamines have been shown to cause cancer in experimental animals; but as we suggested earlier, this does not necessarily mean that humans are similarly susceptible to this carcinogenic potential. Nor is there certain evidence that the nitrites always combine with amines to form nitrosamines in human beings. While the research is under way, the United States Department of Agriculture has reduced the amount of nitrite that can be added to our food.

THE ICE CREAM HEADACHE

Many ice cream lovers experience an intense but brief pain in their throat, head, or face after biting into ice cream or placing a spoonful of ice cream against the back part of the roof of their mouth. The phenomenon has been called the "ice cream headache," but it can happen when any cold substance is similarly positioned. The pain is usually dull and throbbing, frequently radiating throughout the head. Although it can be excruciating, happily the headache lasts only a few minutes.

A complete understanding of this phenomenon is not really known. It is likely to be the result of a physiological response of the warm tissues of the mouth to sudden assault by ice-cold substances. The reason that the pain is felt throughout the head is because the discomfort is referred along the many branches of the fifth and ninth cranial nerves. The fifth cranial nerve carries sensation from the front part of the mouth, whereas the ninth cranial nerve carries sensation from the back of the mouth.

The ice cream headache can be avoided by slowly cooling the mouth. This can be done by allowing small amounts of ice cream to melt in the mouth before devouring the delicacy in globs or scoop by scoop!

There is no doubt that many other foods or chemicals and additives are capable of causing headaches and perhaps more serious medical problems. Some people, including physicians, believe that table salt, for example, provokes headaches. We know that it can aggravate high blood pressure. Continued research will eventually demonstrate that many foods or chemicals currently considered harmless do actually impose considerable health hazards. Legitimate scientific differences of opinion, private interest influence, and governmental administrative delays frequently frustrate the effort to confront these concerns directly, making progress in these areas unfortunately slow.

Chapter **10** "First, Do No Harm"– The Ultimate Responsibility

The most important challenge of any physician is expressed in the Latin phrase *"Primum non nocere"*—"First, do no harm." Before deciding on a treatment or diagnostic program for your illness, a physician's primary commitment is that he/she does not cause more distress than you experienced before help was sought. There is no more important responsibility than this one.

But consider the dilemma. A patient seeks out the assistance of a physician, perhaps begging for relief from painful agony, describing the social or marital woes caused by the distress, and thrusting before the doctor the challenge that he/she can no longer cope. More than once we have heard patients with head pain say, "If you cannot help me, doctor, I will put a gun to my head." And yet, within the limits of our current scientific knowledge, the most reliable and effective treatments for chronic head pain impart at least some potential risk to health. Although progress is rapidly being made in developing safer treatments, such as biofeedback, none at this time can match the speed and efficacy of medication.

Pain relievers are notoriously abused by patients with chronic, recurring pain. It is not uncommon for patients starting with two analgesic tablets every four to six hours for relief to require sixteen to twenty tablets per day months later, seeking out various physicians and druggists to keep the supply available. The consequences can be immense: habituation and addiction, organ (liver, kidney, and stomach) damage, depression, mental dullness, tremors, and much more. Does the benefit justify the risks? Not in the case of analgesics, because analgesics simply *mask* the pain, they do not eliminate it or its course. Analgesics hide pain at best, and current research suggests that an enhanced awareness of that pain may occur when the medicine wears off.

Consider the problem with tranquilizers and antidepressants. Tranquilizers can cause a worsening of existing depression, dull the thinking process a bit, cause sedation, and, when large dosages are taken regularly, induce dependency, posing significant consequences such as seizures and other withdrawal symptoms if the medications are suddenly discontinued. The antidepressants, aside from mild unwanted symptoms such as dry mouth, may lead in certain individuals to heart and blood pressure changes, mental alterations, and other untoward effects. Specific antimigraine medications can alter blood pressure and heart rate, cause changes in circulation, and even induce recurring headaches when overused.

What, then, should the physician do—smile congenially and say, "I'm doing you a favor by not treating you with medications," suggesting instead that you have a psychiatrist assist you in accepting your pain more effectively?

Here is our answer.

First, it must be recognized that, practically speaking, *nothing in our lives*, from the food eaten, the air breathed, the cigarettes smoked, the water imbibed, to the cars driven, *is without considerable, if not greater, health risks than the medicine that a doctor prescribes.* Second, after accepting the fact that at this time in our scientific understanding of pain, the most effective therapies may have some potential hazards associated with their use, a careful and accurate assessment of the need for medication must be carried out. If it is determined that medication absolutely must be used, then potential benefits must be carefully balanced against possible side effects. This important appraisal requires participation by both the doctor and an informed patient. If it is decided to proceed with medical therapy, then you and your doctor must recognize that the real challenge is just beginning.

In practice, most medications, if taken only when necessary and for limited periods of time, actually impose few significant health risks. Unexpected and unforeseeable, and at times tragic, reactions are of course possible. Because science has not yet given us the knowledge to completely understand and control the body and its response to a variety of stimuli, including taking medication, medicine administered by even the most qualified physician will sometimes cause serious reactions. Fortunately, these are relatively unlikely. With dedication to safety by you and your doctor, the risks become minimal.

The physician must carefully and methodically explain when and how to take these drugs, with what other substances and under what circumstances not to take the medications, and educate you about the potential side effects and what to do if these should develop. The doctor must prescribe only limited quantities of the medicines and be aggressively committed to monitoring for the development of those side effects of which you would not otherwise be aware. (Most of these are easily reversible if detected early.) And, as the therapy continues, the physician must seek through innovativeness and ongoing education newer and safer ways of treating you, bringing to your attention new information regarding the drugs that you are taking and newly developed alternative therapies.

For your part, you must be committed to taking the medication precisely as prescribed, being willing to exercise discipline and restraint along with common sense regarding your use of the agents. You must be willing to accept the inconvenience and the cost of appointments with the doctor at regular intervals while on these drugs, and bring to your physician's attention all side effects. You must also allow the doctor to take you off the medications after a while, giving your body a holiday from them, and seek nonmedical therapies to assist you if your discomfort persists or returns.

Both you and your doctor must trust and understand each other, and set reasonable goals for the treatment program. It must be recognized that *total* relief from your discomfort may not be possible within the limits of safe administration of the medications.

In short, for the greatest assurance of safety: use the medicines only when absolutely necessary; employ the lowest dose possible and only for as long as necessary; set reasonable goals for treatment success; and carry out ongoing monitoring and educational communication with your doctor regarding the potential risks, the development of side effects, and alternative therapies. In this way, the concept of "First, do no harm"—your doctor's most important commitment—can be a *living* reality, rather than a tragic irony.

Chapter 11 Finding a Doctor and Helping Yourself

Having severe and recurring headaches imparts a heavy burden on the millions of people plagued by this troubling malady. Common to many of you are feelings of frustration, anger, and desperation. Some see yourselves as conquered victims of headache, who have no choice but to bear the pain for the remainder of your lives.

Despite these feelings of defeat, considerable and sometimes complete relief can be found by most people. To accomplish this, however, you must achieve three critical prerequisites: become sufficiently motivated to help in the effort, find the right doctor for you, and develop a healthy and positive attitude toward yourself.

Finding sufficient motivation to help yourself defeat your headache condition may not be easy. After many years of relentless headaches and the discouragement brought about by many therapeutic failures, you may be resigned to your fate. Nevertheless, becoming motivated to actively participate in your own treatment is essential. Without such motivation, you are deprived of the incentive to persevere during the weeks and perhaps months of working through your headache problem and finding the safest and most effective treatment for you; each headache, each person, is different.

The second prerequisite is finding the right physician. Like all human beings, physicians differ in their personalities, ability, and devotion. The physician who can help you must be able to effectively relate to you, be knowledgeable in headache disorders, be able to inspire trust and confidence from you, and be sufficiently innovative to develop a therapy for your particular needs.

Certain principles should guide you in your choice of doctors. Important signs are the interest and concern your doctor demonstrates when you explain why you seek his/her help. If the doctor shrugs off your headache problem with a "So what else is new, lots of people have headaches" attitude, you would be wise to save your money and seek help elsewhere, because a therapeutically productive relationship between doctor and patient will never be realized. You have the right to insist that your symptoms be taken seriously, and you should not be made to feel foolish for seeking help.

A physician's knowledge regarding headache disorders and the degree of interest in you are often indicated by the amount of detail that the doctor seeks in taking the medical headache history. The medical history must explore many of the characteristic features of the various headache conditions. The medical history represents the most critical component in establishing a correct headache diagnosis, and a successful treatment requires an accurate diagnosis and an assessment of your total emotional as well as medical needs. A doctor who fails to take a detailed history either is not interested in your problem or does not know enough about headaches to ask the important questions. In either case, start looking for a different doctor.

A thorough physical examination must also be performed. Following this, an adequate amount of time should be set aside for your doctor to explain his/her impressions, the diagnostic tests that will be performed, along with the risks that these tests might impose, and the proposed initial treatment, including the possible side effects of all medications that are suggested.

You, as the patient, must have time to ask questions. Arrangements should be made to enable you to maintain regular contact with your doctor while the evaluation and the treatment program are under way, and you must be told what to do should side effects from any part of the treatment develop. When you leave the doctor's office you should have a better understanding of your headaches, and you should know how your doctor will be attempting to help you.

Another very important responsibility of patients, and one that we find often lacking in some that come to see us, is a willingness to accept open-mindedly certain observations regarding their level of stress, anger, or depression. Ironically, patients seem quite willing to accept a diagnosis that suggests that their headaches are rooted in physical disease. But as we have discussed in earlier chapters, many individuals who experience unpleasant symptoms do not have physical disease. Instead, they have overreactive tissue that, in the state of overreactivity, may cause pain. Often, this overreactivity is induced or triggered by emotional distress.

If, after careful consideration, a competent and thoughtful physician suggests the possibility that emotional factors, such as depression, anger, or anxiety, may play a role in your discomfort, it is your responsibility to consider carefully the physician's opinion. You have a right to disagree, and it is possible that the physician is wrong. But in many patients with chronic, unremitting pain, emotional factors capable of triggering physical events *are* present. In order that you be helped, you must assist the physician in designing a treatment program that helps alleviate not only the physical pain but the emotional issues as well. Expecting the physician to do this without your help or insisting that an important component of your mental state be ignored because you consider it irrelevant will surely postpone finding relief.

There are many competent and devoted physicians who successfully treat difficult headache problems. Once you have decided on the physician who deserves your trust and confidence, give that physician and the professionals that work with him/her the benefit of the same patience and tolerance that you expect them to extend to you. Headaches are very stubborn and challenging medical problems. Nevertheless, most patients with headaches can find relief, but it may take time and effort. While it is true that you should never invest blind faith in your physician, you must not enter into a doctor-patient relationship biased against the competence or sincerity of that physician.

If you cannot find the right doctor or if your physician wishes to refer you to a headache specialist, a list of physicians with special interest in headache may be acquired by writing to the National Migraine Foundation, 5214 N. Western Avenue, Chicago, Illinois 60625.

Another challenge that you must face is the development of a healthy, positive, frank, and realistic attitude toward yourself and your headache condition. Here are some suggestions:

You must place yourself and your headaches in proper perspective. Although your headaches may have become part of your existence and have influenced relationships with friends and family, and perhaps even altered your self-image, it is essential that you throw off any negative attitudes. Don't think of yourself as a disabled and beaten person. The very fact that you are seeking answers means that you are making progress in finding a treatment. Actually, just reading this book is itself testimony to your resilience in regard to your headaches; it is a good sign that you have not given up.

Don't be unfair with yourself. You are entitled to personality and character flaws; everyone has them. Perhaps you are at times hostile, tense, insecure, angry, depressed, frightened, and frustrated. None of these, however, sets you apart from any other human being. The trick is to recognize and acknowledge your flaws, modify what you can, and pay special attention to developing your virtues and strengths. Some of the most productive and creative members of our society, past and present, have suffered from headches just like yours. Like them, you too must overcome your headaches' negative influence by refusing to allow headaches to deprive you and those around you of life's pleasures and your creative potential.

We have rarely seen a chronic headache sufferer who could not, if motivated, be more stubborn and resolute than the headache condition. The challenge is to turn these qualities against your headaches instead of against yourself. Once you feel conquered by the pain, you are indeed conquered! Having confidence in your own strength is half the battle; and you can win—not only the battle, but the war!

A fighting attitude favorably balances your virtues against your frailties and your desire to overcome your headaches against their persistent presence. You cannot expect a physician, no matter how capable, to take away what may have become a crutch on which you have learned to lean. You too must join the battle.

Do not see yourself as meek and hurt, desperately searching for help. Instead, place yourself in the company of the many gifted and famous headache sufferers, like Thomas Jefferson, Sigmund Freud, George Bernard Shaw, Chopin, and many others, who refused to let headaches interfere with the contributions they made to society. Do not sell yourself short; most headache victims have not even given themselves a chance. We hope that this book will inspire you to begin, perhaps once again, to find relief.

Appendix: The Brain and Headaches

A SIMPLIFIED ANATOMY AND PHYSIOLOGY OF THE BRAIN

Some of you may wish to understand those parts of the brain's anatomy and function that are relevant to headache disorders. This appendix has been provided for this purpose. At the end of this section you will find a short test which you may use to evaluate your comprehension of this material.

The skull (cranium) is the vault of bone that surrounds and protects the brain. At the base of the skull is a large opening called the foramen magnum. Through this opening the lower end of the brain joins the spinal cord, which continues downward through a canal within the vertebrae (backbones).

The skull is covered by many layers of muscle and skin. Together these compose the tissues of the face and scalp. The muscles surrounding the head overlap muscles coming up from the back and the neck so that the head and the neck are encased in layers of muscle tissue.

An abundant supply of blood vessels and nerves traverses these layers, providing the muscles with the ability to feel pain. Like all muscles throughout the body, the muscles of the scalp, neck, and face can contract. When this contraction is prolonged, the muscles become painful, much like arm and leg pain after strenuous exercise.

The brain is a most remarkable creation. It is composed of billions of small units called cells. Each cell has arm-like extensions called dendrites and axons which carry electrical signals and nourishment into and away from the major portion of the cell, which is called the cell body. Each cell is connected to other brain cells by an intricate network of fibers so that one area of the brain can almost instantly deliver signals to all other areas.

Many of the cells of the brain are "specialized." A specialized cell is capable of carrying out very specific and highly technical functions. For example, a sensory brain cell receives and "feels" the information coming into the brain from various parts of the body. Motor brain cells are specifically programmed to send out directions for motion or action commands to the body organs, like the heart and the gastrointestinal tract, and to the muscles of the body that move the body parts.

Other specialized cells perform additional and complex functions: they store information in memory banks, secrete hormones which stimulate other cells of the brain or body organs to function, and participate in the myriad of activities of the thinking processes.

The brain is organized so that many of the specialized cells are located in precise areas, each devoted to a specific function. The motor areas, for example, are made up of specialized motor cells grouped together in such a way as to provide a "center" for movements of an arm or a leg or other body parts. In a similar way, the sensory portions of the brain represent the area where most sensory information is received, with special locations for vision, hearing, smell, and other senses.

Despite the brain's ability to perceive and register pain and other sensations from the body, ironically the brain itself does not feel pain. In other words, a surgeon's knife does not produce pain when it cuts into brain tissue. However, if the sensory area of your brain representing an arm were damaged, for example, you might not be able to feel pain if your arm were injured.

When an individual suffers from trauma, or injury, to the head and develops head pain as a result, it is not the brain itself that hurts. Instead, the brain perceiving damaged pain-sensitive tissue around the skull and brain is what causes the pain.

The two large lobes of the brain (left and right cerebral [brain] hemispheres) rest upon a stalk of brain tissue called the brain stem. The brain stem has many important functions, and we shall mention a few of them.

One important function of the brain stem is the control of automatic life-sustaining functions. Within the brain stem, for example, are centers for control of heartbeat, breathing, consciousness, and blood pressure. These centers work automatically to keep the body alive. You do not have to think about breathing or making your heart beat in order for these important functions to happen. The brain stem centers carry on without your conscious participation.

Also within the brain stem are centers that control the face, eyes, mouth, and throat. Some of these centers work automatically. Others require conscious participation. For example, when you swallow, the sequence of mouth, tongue, and throat actions is done almost automatically. When you hear a sound coming from one side, you automatically turn your head and eyes in that direction.

Some of the centers in the brain stem serve a sensory function for feeling in the areas about the head and face. Others are purely motor in function.

Emerging from these brain stem centers are nerves that go to the various areas of the head, face, eyes, and mouth. Some of these nerves carry sensory information to the brain stem centers, while others carry motor information from the brain stem to the muscles of the head, face, eyes, and mouth. Because these nerves are responsible for function of the head area, they are called cranial nerves.

Another center within the brain stem is called the activating substance. It is composed of specialized cells whose responsibility it is to act like an electrical generator that sends signals to your cerebral hemispheres to maintain consciousness. If this activating substance fails to perform normally, the hemispheres will cease normal function and you will lose consciousness.

An additional function of the brain stem is to serve as a large conduit transmitting information between the cerebral hemispheres above and the spinal cord below.

It should be clear from this discussion that the brain stem represents the life center for the body. It is here that the control for vital functions (heart, breathing, etc.) resides, and it is here that the "generator" maintaining consciousness is located. All of these important and vital functions are contained in a stalk of brain about one inch in diameter and a few inches long. Even a small area of damage in the brain stem can have a devastating impact on survival.

Resting on the back of the brain stem is a portion of brain called the cerebellum. The cerebellum is responsible for control of balance and coordination. Many of the medications used to treat pain can temporarily impair the function of the cerebellum, and when this occurs, incoordination and imbalance result. The cerebellum is very sensitive to the effects of alcohol, and it is because of this sensitivity that staggering and incoordination follow the excessive drinking of intoxicating beverages.

The brain stem continues downward through the neck to become the spinal cord. The spinal cord is located outside the skull, extracranially, and runs down your back. Like the brain stem, the spinal cord serves as a conduit for entering and exiting nerves and their communication to and from the body and the cerebral hemispheres.

Motor fibers originating in the cerebral hemispheres and going to the arms travel down through the brain stem into the spinal cord and exit from the spinal cord in the neck region. They then go through the shoulder region and into the arms. Sensory information from the hands and arms will enter the spinal cord in the neck region and then run up through the brain stem, eventually finding its way to the arm and hand sensory cell area of the cerebral hemispheres. The nerves that enter and exit from the spinal cord are called spinal, or peripheral, nerves.

The spinal cord is about the same diameter as a medium-sized carrot, a little more than one-half inch. Like all other nerve tissue, the spinal cord is very fragile. For protection, the spinal cord and its nerves are enclosed within a tunnel formed by many vertebrae, the backbones. The vertebrae do not move freely because there would be great risk of tearing the very fragile spinal cord and damaging the entering and exiting nerves. To help prevent the vertebrae from moving excessively, they are surrounded by a covering of muscles and ligaments that firmly hold the vertebrae in line.

The brain and spinal cord are covered by layers of tissue called the meninges. The nerves and blood vessels entering and exiting the brain stem and spinal cord must go through the meninges. This tissue is very sensitive to pain, and any irritation or inflammation can be a source of discomfort, felt as a headache.

The nerve fibers are like small electrical cables containing the sensory and motor fibers going to and coming from the brain stem or the spinal cord. As mentioned earlier, the nerves that emerge from or enter the brain stem are called cranial nerves because they influence the head (cranial) area, while those that enter and exit from the spinal cord are called the spinal, or peripheral, nerves. There are twelve paired cranial nerves that serve motor and sensory functions of the head, face, and special automatic vital functions. There are about thirty paired spinal nerves and these serve the rest of the body.

Certain of the nerves are particularly important in a discussion of headaches. The fifth cranial nerve, also called the trigeminal nerve, is the major sensory nerve carrying feeling information from most portions of the face and scalp. The fifth cranial nerve also carries feeling from the front portion of the tissue that covers the brain, the meninges.

In addition to the fifth cranial nerve, the neck, or cervical, nerves are important to headache problems because these nerves carry pain sensation from the neck and the back of the head into the spinal cord and then up to the cerebral hemispheres.

A very important concept related to pain and thus to headache problems is called the phenomenon of referred pain. By virtue of referred pain a discomfort or irritation originating in one area may actually be perceived as pain coming from another location. There are many examples of this. Perhaps the most well known example is that during a heart attack, pain originating in the heart may be "referred," or displaced, and thus perceived as coming from the left arm.

When considering headache problems, an understanding of the concept of referred pain is particularly important. As pointed out earlier, the fifth cranial nerve carries pain sensation from most regions of the face, eyes, forehead, sinuses, mouth, and even coverings of the brain. As a result of referred pain, any irritation or abnormality in any of these areas can be perceived as pain coming from another area. Thus, pain from a dental problem could be experienced as pain over the forehead or in an eye. Pain from a tumor irritating the meninges could be felt as pain in the temples or in an eye. Similarly, pain from irritation of the spinal nerves of the neck from arthritis, for example, could be referred along the upper spinal nerves and be felt as pain in the top or back of the head or from behind an ear.

The reason for referred pain is complex and not fully understood. In general, it is the result of a single nerve or part of the spinal cord carrying or receiving information from more than one location. When information from one of these areas is perceived in the sensory area of the cerebral hemispheres, it is sometimes "misperceived" as coming from somewhere else.

Within the center of the cerebral hemispheres is a series of interconnecting canals called ventricles. These canals continue downward from the cerebral hemispheres into the brain stem. Inside the ventricles is a fluid called the cerebrospinal fluid, which is a clear liquid produced by specialized cells and blood vessels that line the ventricles. The cerebrospinal fluid bathes, cushions, and brings nourishment to the brain. Cerebrospinal fluid exits the canal system through openings in the brain stem and then enters spaces between the layers of the meninges. It then circulates around the brain and the spinal cord. When a spinal tap is performed, the cerebrospinal fluid circulating between the layers of the meninges in the lower portion of the lower spinal cord is removed for evaluation.

Within the bones of the skull are spaces that are lined by special mucous-secreting cells. These spaces are called sinuses. The fifth cranial nerve is responsible for carrying sensation from the sinuses. These sinuses can become inflamed and infected. When severe, these processes can result in blockage. Pain arising from the sinuses can be referred elsewhere along the course of the fifth cranial nerve. In the same way, pain from other areas served by the fifth cranial nerve can be felt in the sinus area, giving the false impression that the sinuses are the source of the discomfort.

Advertisements selling sinus headache remedies conveniently overlook this fact, as well as many others. The commercials infer that if you have pain over your sinuses, you have sinus problems. It is estimated that less than at best only 10 percent of people who suffer pain over their sinuses actually have sinus trouble. (See Chapter 5.)

Let us now leave anatomy and briefly discuss the physiology of the brain.

Physiology is a term referring to the way the body functions. While no one truly understands the complex mechanism of the brain, it is well established that, in part, the brain functions by virtue of electrical currents that travel from cell to cell within the cerebral hemispheres and up and down the brain stem, spinal cord, and nerves. These electrical currents are generated by the action of chemical substances upon the cells. These substances are called neurotransmitters.

Although there are various types of neurotransmitters, those that seem most important to headache problems are called amines. Amines are important for proper brain and nerve activity and are critical to various important functions, including sleeping, controlling blood pressure, heart rate, and even for determining various moods. An overabundance of amines, a deficiency of them, or other abnormality of the amines is related to a number of important neurological and psychiatric disorders, such as Parkinson's disease, depression, schizophrenia, Huntington's disease, and migraine headaches.

TERMS AND CONCEPTS

The language of medicine has developed over centuries, and many of the phrases and terms used today reflect their Greek or Latin origin.

The following are some of the terms and medical concepts, in alphabetical order, which are relevant to the subject of headaches. You will have encountered these during your reading, and this list will serve as a concise review of them.

Amines—Biological substances that are necessary for brain and blood vessel function. Some amines are found in food; others are produced by the body. The amines are very important; they influence mood, behavior, and the degree of constriction or dilation of blood vessels. Abnormalities of the amines cause various diseases.

Analgesics—Medications that reduce the perception of pain by raising your pain threshold. Analgesics do not cure the cause of the pain but simply cover it up or mask it. Analgesics range from simple analgesics (like aspirin) to narcotic analgesics (like morphine).

Antidepressants—Medications designed to raise the spirits of seriously depressed people. Antidepressants work by elevating the level of those amines that are deficient in various mood and behavioral abnormalities. Antidepressants may also have a beneficial effect on certain headache problems even when depression is not present.

Chronic—Refers to anything that is of long-standing duration. For example, a chronic headache condition is one that has occurred frequently over a period of many years.

Extracranial—Refers to anything outside the skull. The scalp, for example, is an extracranial structure.

Inflammation—This term refers to the expected response of living tissue to irritation or injury. When tissue is assaulted, there occurs a rush of various body substances and blood cells into the affected area. This results in redness, swelling, and warmth—a process called inflammation. Very often the inflammation following an injury or an allergic reaction is more responsible for the discomfort than is the initial injury or allergy.

Intracranial—Refers to anything inside the skull. The brain is an intracranial structure.

Motor—Refers to moving or causing motion. The motor area of the brain and the motor nerves carry movement commands to the muscles that affect the motor, or movement, activity.

Muscle contraction or spasm—Muscles throughout the body can become cramped by becoming contracted in spasm. Muscle contraction may occur in response to injury, fatigue of the muscles, or emotional stress. Like inflammation, muscle contraction may cause more discomfort than the injury by which it is triggered.

Over-the-counter drugs—Refers to nonprescription drugs or medications that can be purchased without a doctor's prescription. Popular over-the-counter drugs include headache and sinus headache medications and cold preparations.

Pain threshold—Refers to the level of your sensitivity to pain. In effect, it is the degree of discomfort that a sensation must cause in order for you to perceive it as painful. Pain threshold varies from person to person and even within the same individual from one moment to another. Pain threshold can be altered by various factors, including biological events as well as emotional ones. Depression and irritability can lower pain threshold so that a less intense stimulus will be perceived as painful. Analgesics and emotional contentment raise pain threshold so that it takes a more intense stimulation to be felt as painful.

Paraspinal muscles—Refers to muscles located just to the side (para-) of the vertebral spine (the bumps down the center of your back). The cervical (neck) paraspinal muscles contract in response to many factors, including arthritis in the neck region and emotional upset. The pain from this contraction is often perceived as a headache.

Photophobia—Refers to an uncomfortable visual sensitivity to light. Photophobia often accompanies migraine headaches.

Placebo—A drug or treatment that has no known medical benefit other than that associated with the suggestion that it will work.

Placebo effect or response—Refers to the beneficial effect that a placebo medication will have when given to certain individuals. It is estimated that more than 40 percent of individuals with headaches who are given a placebo treatment will initially experience an improvement of their symptoms.

Scotoma—A blind spot of varying size and shape that can occur within the field of vision. Scotomas are sometimes present during migraine headaches. When a scotoma is present, areas of your vision are effectively blurred or blinded.

Sensory—A term referring to a sensation or feeling. A sensory nerve carries feeling information to the sensory portion of the brain.

Syndrome—A group of symptoms often occurring together and resulting from a particular abnormal condition or disease. The migraine syndrome, for example, refers to the group of symptoms, including pain, nausea and vomiting, and photophobia, that might occur during a migraine headache.

Tranquilizers—Medications that calm and lessen anxiety and emotional tension. Side effects can include sleepiness, light-headedness, and a sense of imbalance and incoordination.

Vasoconstriction—A term describing the narrowing of blood vessels. (Vaso- is a prefix referring to blood vessels, i.e., veins and arteries.)

Vasodilation—A term that is the opposite of vasoconstriction and refers to the widening, or distension, of a blood vessel.

A QUIZ

For daring readers who would like to test their understanding of the material in this book, the following is a true-and-false quiz that you may want to take. You may be surprised at how much you have learned if you have read this book carefully.

	True	False
1. Referred pain is a discomfort that is felt somewhere other than where the irritation occurs.	——	——

	True	False
2. An analgesic has curative as well as pain-relieving ability.	____	____
3. The brain itself feels no pain when directly injured.	____	____
4. Nerve fibers that carry feeling information *to* the brain are called motor nerves.	____	____
5. The spinal cord is very durable and can easily withstand stretching and twisting movements.	____	____
6. The cranial nerve responsible for feeling pain around the face and the head is the fifth cranial nerve.	____	____
7. A placebo is a medication with important curative properties.	____	____
8. Vasodilation means nerve widening.	____	____
9. Pain threshold refers to the intensity of a stimulation necessary for it to be felt as painful.	____	____
10. Pain threshold cannot be altered by mood and emotions.	____	____
11. The cerebellum is important for visual perception.	____	____
12. The meninges are pain-sensitive structures covering the brain.	____	____
13. The cells that control movement are called motor cells.	____	____
14. Pain originating in the neck may be perceived as coming from behind an ear.	____	____
15. The vertebrae are designed to allow free and maximum movement in all directions.	____	____
16. Amines serve as neurotransmitters and assist in brain cell function.	____	____
17. Generally speaking, inflammation is not painful.	____	____
18. Physiology means the study of body function.	____	____
19. Pain over a sinus may be coming from the mouth.	____	____
20. Most headaches over the forehead are due to disease of the sinuses.	____	____

True False

21. The function of the cerebellum may be temporarily impaired by certain drugs, like tranquilizers or alcohol, resulting in imbalance and incoordination. ___ ___

22. A chronic headache condition is one that has just developed recently. ___ ___

23. A scotoma is a type of brain tumor. ___ ___

24. Many headache sufferers will experience at least a temporary beneficial response from medication that possesses no active ingredients. ___ ___

25. Over-the-counter drugs are those that do not require a prescription. ___ ___

26. An amine may influence your mood, sleep, and the degree of dilation and constriction of your blood vessels. ___ ___

27. Muscles around the neck and scalp may contract and cause headaches. ___ ___

28. Photophobia refers to the visual discomfort to light that may occur during a migraine headache. ___ ___

29. Muscle contraction or spasm can result from emotional factors. ___ ___

30. The brain stem contains centers responsible for automatic breathing. ___ ___

An answer key follows.

Answer Key

1. True.
2. False. Analgesics do not cure; they only raise pain threshold.
3. True.
4. False. Motor nerves carry information *from* the brain; sensory nerves carry information to it.
5. False. The spinal cord is very fragile and thus needs the strong support of the vertebrae and ligaments.

6. True.
7. False. It is an inert substance thought to be effective primarily because of suggestion.
8. False. Vasodilation refers to blood vessel widening, not nerve widening.
9. True.
10. False. Pain threshold can definitely be influenced by emotion.
11. False. The cerebellum is important for balance and coordination.
12. True.
13. True.
14. True.
15. False. Only limited movement is allowed, thus protecting the spinal cord and also supporting the trunk of the body.
16. True.
17. False. Inflammation is most certainly painful.
18. True.
19. True.
20. False. Ten percent or less of patients with pain over the forehead actually suffer from disease of the sinuses.
21. True.
22. False. Chronic headaches are those present for many months or years.
23. False. A scotoma is a "blind spot" in the field of vision.
24. True.
25. True.
26. True.
27. True.
28. True.
29. True.
30. True.

INDEX

Abdominal muscles, 103
Abortive treatment, 28-29, 80-83
Acetaminophen, 31, 36, 37, 80, 112, 132, 148
  with aspirin, 32
  in Excedrin tablets, 32-33
Acetylsalicylic acid, 31
Acupuncture, 38, 47-48
Airplane travel, 73
Alcohol, 69, 128
  amines in, 195
  hangover, 165-66
  for relaxation, 46-47
  sensitivity to, 122, 123-24
  and tranquilizers, 39
Alice in Wonderland syndrome, 58, 59, 98
Alice's Adventures in Wonderland (Carroll), 16, 58, 98
Allergic sinus headache, 131, 133-34
American Association for the Study of Headaches, 47
American Heart Journal, 197
American Journal of Psychiatry, 192
Amines, 55, 216
  in food, 193-95
Amitriptyline, 43, 83-84, 113

Anacin, 33-36, 157, 191, 192
  ingredients, effects, dose, and alternative to, 34-35
Analgesics, 29-38, 102, 112, 114, 116, 142, 150, 153, 202
  advantages of, 29
  brain and, 38
  dose (drug X compared to drug Y), 30
  for migraine, 79-80
  narcotic, 30, 38, 80, 113
  over-the-counter, 30, 31-38
  potency, side effects and cost, 30
  problems caused by use of, 29-30
  See also Aspirin; names of analgesics
Anger, 137, 141
Angiogram, 95
Antacids, 33
Anticoagulants, 31
Antidepressants, 39, 42-44, 83, 112, 113, 142, 156, 202
  tricyclic, 43-44, 160
Antihistamines, 30, 36, 37, 84, 133, 160
Antinauseants, 30, 80, 82, 83
Anxiety, 20, 24, 39, 41, 42, 46, 137, 141, 152, 154, 162, 163
"Anxiety or Caffeinism: A Diagnostic Dilemma" (Greden), 192

225